Research on Social Work and Disasters

Research on Social Work and Disasters

Calvin L. Streeter
Susan A. Murty
Editors

Routledge
Taylor & Francis Group
NEW YORK AND LONDON

Research on Social Work and Disasters has also been published as *Journal of Social Service Research*, Volume 22, Numbers 1/2 1996.

First published 1996 by The Haworth Press, Inc.

This edition published 2012 by Routledge
605 Third Avenue, New York, NY 10017
2 Park Square, Milton Park, Abingdon, Oxon OX14 4RN

Routledge is an imprint of the Taylor & Francis Group, an informa business

Library of Congress Cataloging-in-Publication Data

Research on social work and disasters / Calvin L. Streeter, Susan A. Murty, editors.
p. cm.
"Has . . . been published as Journal of social service research, volume 22, numbers 1/2, 1996"–T.p. verso.
Includes bibliographical references and index.
ISBN 0-7890-0028-8 (hbk. : alk. paper). – ISBN 0-7890-0303-1 (pbk. : alk. paper)
1. Disaster relief–Research–United States. 2. Social service–Research–United States. I. Streeter, Calvin L. II. Murty, Susan A.

HV553.R39 1996
363.34'8'0973–dc21 96-40923
CIP

ISBN 13: 978-0-7890-0028-6 (hbk)

Research on Social Work and Disasters

CONTENTS

ABOUT THE EDITORS

Calvin L. Streeter, PhD, is Associate Professor and Chair of the Administration and Planning Concentration in the School of Social Work at the University of Texas at Austin. He has been a member of the faculty at the University of Texas since 1989 and teaches courses on human services management, program planning and evaluation, community organization, and research methods. His current research interests include disaster preparedness and community response to crisis, school social work and dropout prevention, and innovations in human services delivery systems. He is a member of the Board of Directors for the Association for Community Organization and Social Administration (ACOSA). Dr. Streeter's recent work has been published in the journal *Social Work* and in the book *Total Quality Management in the Social Services.* He is also co-author of the forthcoming *Disasters and Development: International Disaster Planning.*

Susan A. Murty, PhD, is Assistant Professor in the School of Social Work at the University of Iowa. Her areas of research include interorganizational relations, rural and regional service delivery, and network analysis. She is President of the National Rural Social Work Caucus and serves on the advisory board of the journal *Human Services in the Rural Environment*. Dr. Murty is a member of the National Association for Rural Mental Health, the National Association of Social Workers, the Council on Social Work Education, and the Association for Community Organization and Social Administration (ACOSA). Her recent work on network analysis and disaster services was published in the *Journal of Applied Social Sciences* and the *American Journal of Community Psychology.*

Introduction

The idea of this special volume was developed by David Gillespie, who has been contributing to research on interorganizational coordination for disaster preparedness for many years. He suggested that we take on the project of co-editing this volume and has supported and encouraged us all along the way.

The social work profession has a historical tradition of responding generously when disasters strike. The profession has been called on to respond more and more frequently in recent years as the number of natural and technological disasters has increased and the size of the populations affected has also grown. Recovery from Hurricanes Hugo, Andrew, and Iniki is far from complete even now and the disastrous hurricane season of 1995 suggests that we should be prepared for more severe hurricanes in the coming years. The Loma Prieta and Northridge Earthquakes gave us an indication of the magnitude of disaster we can expect in the many parts of the country which are vulnerable to seismic activity. The Mid-West floods in 1993 left many homeless and recovery is slow.

Because larger populations now live and work on land vulnerable to various hazards, natural disasters can be expected to affect more people each year. But the technological or human-made disasters add to the deadly effects of natural disasters. Not only do toxic and nuclear waste create new hazards of their own, but the effects of natural disasters on humans are worsened when technological hazards are unleashed following hurricanes, tornadoes, storms, floods,

---

[Haworth co-indexing entry note]: "Introduction." Streeter, Calvin L. and Susan A. Murty. Co-published simultaneously in *Journal of Social Service Research* (The Haworth Press, Inc.) Vol. 22, No. 1/2, 1996, pp. 1-6; and: *Research on Social Work and Disasters* (ed: Calvin L. Streeter and Susan A. Murty) The Haworth Press, Inc., 1996, pp. 1-6. Single or multiple copies of this article are available for a fee from The Haworth Document Delivery Service [1-800-342-9678, 9:00 a.m. - 5:00 p.m. (EST). E-mail address: getinfo@haworth.com].

and earthquakes. In the next decades, the social work profession will be stretched to its limits as it attempts to respond to growing human needs in the wake of disaster. For these reasons, it is essential that social workers develop effective strategies for dealing with these growing needs.

At a time when research on disasters is so urgently needed, it is encouraging to note the work being carried out by an increasing number of researchers in the fields of social work and the social sciences. Traumatic stress and stress debriefing now receive considerable attention from researchers and practitioners in the fields of social work, psychology, and psychiatry. This work is being incorporated into research on disasters and emergencies. The newly formed Symposium on Disaster and Traumatic Stress at the Council on Social Work Education meetings is one indication of the growing importance of research on disasters. The annual workshop held by the Natural Hazards Research and Applications Information Center at the University of Colorado at Boulder is another. Clearly the importance of disaster research is becoming more widely recognized. This special collection features examples of recent research on disasters chosen to illustrate a variety of types of disasters, theoretical approaches, methodologies, and levels of analysis.

The research presented is consistent with the tradition and mission of the social work profession in several ways. In the first place, all the papers focus on the interaction between individuals and various aspects of their environment. They deal with social problems at multiple levels: the individual and family, the organizational and the interorganizational network, the community, and the societal and policy levels. While striving to meet high standards for scientific research, these studies nevertheless uphold the mission of social work to advocate for those who are experiencing unusual hardships. The implications drawn from the research are consistent in suggesting the responsibility of society to care for vulnerable populations and to share the burdens caused by catastrophic events.

However, these articles do more than uphold the historical traditions of social work. They present innovative work focusing on disasters, an area of research that has been neglected by the profession in the past. They use advanced quantitative and qualitative research methodologies. In addition to addressing effective strategies for responding in the aftermath of particular disasters, the papers in this volume also suggest significant ways in which the social work profession can become involved in prevention, mitigation, and preparedness activities.

The first article is written by Michael Zakour of the School of Social Work at Tulane University. This paper provides an overview of disaster research and the role of the social work profession in relation to disaster. Zakour is uniquely qualified to present this paper since he was the original organizer of the Disaster and Traumatic Stress Symposium at the annual program meetings of the Council on Social Work Education. In addition to pursuing his own research on volunteers and organizations responding to disasters, Zakour has been active in promoting disaster research among social workers.

The second article is written by Elane Nuehring of the School of Social Work at Barry University and Sally Dodds of the Department of Psychiatry and Behavioral Sciences at the University of Miami. This paper offers a "blueprint for research readiness." Nuehring and Dodds propose strategies to overcome barriers to carrying out disaster research in schools of social work. The paper presents a theoretical stress model which will be useful to many disaster researchers. It discusses a range of important issues related to disaster research including funding, ethics, research design, methodology, and measurement. The authors suggest ways in which schools of social work can carry out advanced preparation for research on disasters and work in partnership with other schools so as to be able to assist researchers in the immediate aftermath of disaster events.

The next two articles are examples of the type of research proposed by Nuehring and Dodds. Both are research projects carried out at schools of social work and both provide social work students with opportunities to learn about disasters and to develop research skills. In this way, disasters can be used to provide a laboratory experience for students. Both papers focus on response to natural disasters. Both show how such research can be used to guide efforts to protect the most vulnerable individuals and communities from the impact of disasters.

The third article is written by Paul Sundet and Joanne Mermelstein of the School of Social Work at the University of Missouri at Columbia. This paper compares case studies of eight small river towns in the Midwest which were severely affected by the floods of 1993. Sundet and Mermelstein apply a theoretical model based on crisis theory both at the micro level of individual response and the macro level of community response to traumatic stress. They show how data collection for this study was incorporated into a graduate social work class on community processes. The community is the unit of analysis in this research. The paper explores factors associated with the ability of certain of these towns to survive after the floods.

The fourth article is written by Andrew Cherry of the School of Social Work at Barry University and Mary Elizabeth Cherry of the Biscayne Institute in Miami, Florida. This paper uses a social action research approach which is consistent with the traditional focus of the social work profession on advocacy for vulnerable populations. It reports on the effects of another natural disaster, Hurricane Andrew, on the homeless population of South Florida. It uses an innovative methodology to estimate the size of the homeless population. The data were collected by interviewing teams made up of one graduate social work student and one person who had previously experienced homelessness. The findings of this research were successfully used to advocate for continued relief efforts and to influence policy on behalf of the homeless affected by Hurricane Andrew.

The next two articles report on research on the human-made or technological disasters which are becoming more frequent and having greater impact as advanced technologies become more widely used. Although strikingly different in methodology, these two papers share a common concern with the impact of technological disasters on vulnerable populations with little access to power. Both papers also address the special problems faced by rural as opposed to urban residents.

The fifth article is written by Hussein Soliman of the School of Social Work at Southern Illinois University at Carbondale. Soliman applies a social process model of research to a case study of a rural community which was affected by a long history of pollution. The paper focuses on the effects of the pollution on individual residents and the community as a whole. It documents the stages of response and confrontation which the community went through over the years as it struggled to cope with the effects of toxic waste in its river.

The sixth article is written by Mary Rogge of the College of Social Work at the University of Tennessee at Knoxville. This paper uses an advanced quantitative methodology to study the factors associated with exposure to toxic chemicals. The study uses data from the Environmental Protection Agency on toxics released to the air from industrial and commercial manufacturing facilities. It uses a conceptual approach based on theories of social justice and distributive justice. The paper shows how demographic characteristics, income levels, and racial composition are associated with social vulnerability to toxic risk.

The last article is written by Charles Faupel of the Department of Sociology, Anthropology, and Social Work at Auburn University and Jack Kartez of the Environmental Science and Policy Program at the University of Southern Maine. Faupel and Kartez use a theoretical approach derived from resource dependency theory applied to interorganizational coordination. Using multivariate analysis, this paper focuses on community education as a strategy for improving preparedness and for mitigating the effects of disaster. The paper points out the important role which local government plays in these efforts. It suggests that it would be effective for social workers to collaborate in local community hazard education efforts with the professional emergency managers and city planners who are often engaged in such activities.

We are grateful for the opportunity to work with the authors who have contributed to this special collection and we commend David Gillespie for his work in promoting disaster research in the field of social work. We hope that this volume will serve to focus the attention of the profession on disasters as a field of practice and encourage researchers to pursue the lines of inquiry which have been presented here. By adding to the knowledge base about disasters, researchers can help to contribute to effective social work practice to prevent, mitigate, and reduce the impact of disasters nationally and world-wide. We hope to see many more papers on disaster research appear. This compendium should be the beginning of a fine new tradition in the social work profession.

Calvin L. Streeter
School of Social Work
University of Texas at Austin

Susan A. Murty
School of Social Work
University of Iowa

Disaster Research in Social Work

Michael J. Zakour

SUMMARY. Disaster research in social work has deep roots in the profession's history of disaster relief, social work's mission to create resources and make them accessible to people, and the profession's service to vulnerable populations. Social workers have important and unique contributions to make to disaster research through their expertise in ecological approaches, prevention, stress and coping, and promoting change in micro and macro systems. Disaster research in social work borrows primarily from psychology and sociology, and is conducted in clinical, organizational, and community contexts. Further social work research on disaster promises improved theory, measurement, and practice in situations of collective stress. *[Article copies available for a fee from The Haworth Document Delivery Service: 1-800-342-9678. E-mail address: getinfo@haworth.com]*

The social work profession has historically provided relief during disasters, and disaster intervention and research is highly consistent

---

Michael J. Zakour, PhD, is Assistant Professor, Tulane University School of Social Work, New Orleans, LA 70118.

The author acknowledges the helpful suggestions and comments of the editors, Calvin L. Streeter and Susan A. Murty, on drafts of this paper.

This material is partially based on work supported by the Louisiana Board of Regents through the Louisiana Education Quality Support Fund (LEQSF) under Grant Number LEQSF(RF/1995-98)-RD-A-43 at Tulane University. Any opinions, findings, and conclusions or recommendations expressed in this article are those of the author and do not necessarily reflect the views of the Louisiana Board of Regents or the LEQSF program.

[Haworth co-indexing entry note]: "Disaster Research in Social Work." Zakour, Michael J. Co-published simultaneously in *Journal of Social Service Research* (The Haworth Press, Inc.) Vol. 22, No. 1/2, 1996, pp. 7-25; and: *Research on Social Work and Disasters* (ed: Calvin L. Streeter and Susan A. Murty) The Haworth Press, Inc., 1996, pp. 7-25. Single or multiple copies of this article are available for a fee from The Haworth Document Delivery Service [1-800-342-9678, 9:00 a.m. - 5:00 p.m. (EST). E-mail address: getinfo@haworth.com].

with social work's mission. Social service organizations with substantial social worker involvement are an important part of disaster services (Gillespie, 1991). Based on social work's history of disaster relief, the profession's mission to create resources and make them accessible to people, and the profession's service to disadvantaged populations, disaster research is being conducted by social workers at micro and macro levels. Social work disaster research promises improved theory, measurement, and practice in situations of crisis, traumatic stress, and collective suffering.

Disasters are crisis situations, involving more than one household, which are precipitated by natural agents, technological accidents, environmental contamination, transportation accidents, mass violence, and the sudden death of key individuals in an organization. Social work research into disasters seeks to improve our understanding of mitigation, preparedness, response, and recovery from these situations of traumatic stress and collective suffering. Increased understanding helps improve social work interventions in disaster, and better educates social workers for effective disaster intervention. Research knowledge is important to social work clinicians, managers, and policy practitioners, many of whom play major roles in disaster relief services.

Both natural and man-made disasters are rapidly increasing in frequency and severity, with large segments of the total population in need of relief services. With global population growth, disadvantaged populations are increasing in areas vulnerable to disaster and ecological collapse. As Dodds and Nuehring indicate further on, substantial population movement into coastal areas has increased the vulnerability of the U.S. population to natural disasters such as storms, hurricanes, and floods. Most states in the United States are vulnerable to earthquakes.

HISTORY OF DISASTER SOCIAL WORK

Historically, social work has placed its primary emphasis on emergency services, especially in wartime, disaster, and crisis situations requiring a volunteer cadre. Though social work has always played a central role in disasters, little recognition of this has existed inside or outside the profession (Siporin, 1987). Health and mental health services in wartime represent one of the earliest activities of the profession. Encouraged by the successes of medical social workers during the Civil War, social workers and public health officials organized the public to remove environmental causes of ill health, including polluted drinking water, garbage, crowded tenement dwellings, and industrial hazards (Trattner, 1994). In the health and mental health movements, social workers mobilized officials, lay persons, volunteers, concerned groups, and constituents to prevent disease and disability through improving the environment. Social work military support services continue to the present day through involvement in the American Red Cross, and environmental pollution continues to challenge social workers to assist communities threatened by exposure to hazards (Rogge, 1995).

Volunteers and Emergency Services

An early focus of social work was the provision of volunteer emergency relief for household destitution, urban unrest, epidemics, and social dislocation (Trattner, 1994). Charity Organization Societies provided relief services in the Chicago fire of 1871 and the San Francisco earthquake and fire of 1906 (Siporin, 1987). In the aftermath of Hurricane Betsy in Louisiana, at least one social work school temporarily suspended educational operations and volunteered faculty and students for the relief effort (Speizman & Lloyd, 1965).

These earlier social work relief efforts show the importance of combining volunteer action and professional expertise to provide emergency services. The relief efforts also reflect social work's emphasis on mobilizing diverse community groups, and coordinating these volunteer and professional groups to improve services for suffering populations. Just as interagency coordination promised improved services during the Charity Organization Society era, improved coordination holds great promise for improving emergency relief today. This emphasis on coordination in disaster settings is highly consistent with the social work mission to bolster resources to help people cope with crisis situations, and to provide links among resource systems to make them more accessible to people (Minahan & Pincus, 1977).

THE SOCIAL WORK MISSION AND DISASTERS

As the history of the profession suggests, disaster research and intervention furthers the mission of social work. Practice and research in disaster social services advances the goals of the profession through (a) providing needed resources for disadvantaged and vulnerable populations, (b) preventing serious health and mental health consequences, (c) linking individuals and resource systems, (d) linking various resource systems to make them more accessible to people, and (e) changing micro and macro systems to promote improved client welfare.

Vulnerable Populations

Social work, among the helping professions, is particularly concerned with improving the well-being and welfare of disadvantaged and vulnerable populations (Minahan & Pincus, 1977). Older persons, children, the disabled, less educated persons, and particularly low-income persons are more vulnerable to disaster, and less able to respond and recover in disaster. Because people of color are disproportionately of lower socioeconomic status, they too are more vulnerable to disaster's effects. Individuals and populations at-risk for other biopsychosocial problems are at greatly increased risk from disaster, and these individuals make up a very large percentage of victims suffering from disaster's long-term effects (Smith, North, & Price, 1988).

Paralleling increased individual vulnerability, disadvantaged or economically depressed communities are more vulnerable to long-term deterioration from disasters. These groups and communities disproportionately suffer from Post-Traumatic Stress Disorder and other mental health problems, disability, family breakups, lack of access to relief services, and community disintegration (Siporin, 1987). Social work with vulnerable individuals and groups emphasizes a strengths-based approach, which disaster intervention and research promotes through a stress and coping framework.

Prevention

Consistent with social work's focus on the individual in the social environment, the profession aims to prevent illness through promoting a healthy environment for people (Trattner, 1994). Berger and Kelly (1993) propose that the notion of environment should be extended to all biosystems. This broader definition of environment would direct the profession to improve human welfare by mitigating global disasters, including worldwide ecological collapse. Disaster mitigation and preparedness are primary prevention activities, and both efforts require social work expertise. This expertise includes knowledge of the health and mental health effects of severe stress, knowledge of trauma's impact on families, and expertise in agency and program coordination. The most effective means to communicate evacuation warnings to non-English-speaking, disabled, or older populations is an additional aspect of social work's expertise in prevention.

Many of the approaches to disaster relief are preventive approaches. Debriefing for traumatic stress reactions in disasters uses group work methods, and aims at preventing more serious stress reactions (Armstrong, Lund, McWright, & Tichenor, 1995). Response and recovery prevent much more serious, long-term, and intractable psychosocial problems including mental illness, physical illness, violence, and substance abuse. Intervention also helps prevent serious family, group, organizational, and community disruption. The social work public education role in disaster aims at educating people through disseminating information to social networks through gatekeepers, leaders, and natural helpers (Coulter & Noss, 1988; Dufka, 1988).

Access to Services

Social workers strive to improve people's access to resources and services by creating links between people and resource systems, and linking various resource systems (Minahan & Pincus, 1977). Social workers in disaster seek to promote access to relief resources for people through outreach, case finding, advocacy, and brokering. These social work roles in disaster are being increasingly emphasized by the American Red Cross in provision of disaster services.

Social workers also humanize relief services, programs, and organizations, making them more user-friendly for disaster victims. These social work activities are particularly beneficial to vulnerable populations, whose extended families may lack the resources to provide informal relief, and who have particular difficulty accessing formal relief services (Bolin, 1988). In the case of man-made technological disasters, communities may be blocked from accessing coping resources through public and media campaigns waged by the industries which cause the disaster. As Soliman suggests, social workers can help these victim communities through community development, advocacy, outreach, and brokering actions.

Service Coordination

Service coordination has been an important social work role since the Charity Organization Societies, and it is a critical activity for social service organizations during times of financial restraint (Streeter, Gillespie, Sherraden, & Zakour, 1986). During disaster, coordination of programs and services facilitates an effective response. Coordination is also necessary for rapid and timely provision of services, to prevent what Erickson (1976) calls the "second disaster." Coordination is currently a central concern for the International Decade for Natural Disaster Reduction (IDNDR), which originated in a 1990 United Nations resolution signed by 155 member nations (Gillespie, 1991).

Change at Micro and Macro Levels

Change at both micro and macro levels is a central objective for social workers. This objective is reflected in social work in disasters. Dodds and Nuehring, in this collection, state that social workers help to make services more accessible to people, ensure that vulnerable populations receive coordinated services, and help prevent deterioration in victims' health, mental health, and overall functioning. Social workers help families, groups, organizations, and communities prepare for and process the traumatic stress of disasters. Social workers change organizations, interorganizational networks, communities, and larger social structures to improve disaster preparedness and mitigation. Community social structure may be changed by institutionalizing the gemeinschaft altruistic community, so that it becomes a permanent part of the gesellschaft, bureaucratic recovery phase (Siporin, 1987). According to Soliman, change is needed at both micro and macro levels because disaster's effects reverberate over time from the individual to the organizational and societal levels.

CURRENT AND FUTURE TRENDS IN DISASTER RESEARCH

Scope of Social Work Involvement in Disaster

Disasters are causing an unprecedented rise in demand for social work services. Examples of this increased demand are Hurricane Andrew which left 350,000 homeless, the Mexico City earthquake which left 500,000 homeless and 100,000 without jobs (Dufka, 1988), and the Great Flood of 1993 which, as Sundet and Mermelstein report, inundated over 70 communities and placed tens of thousands of families at risk for physical and mental health problems (Kreuger, Stretch, & Hatfield, 1995). Projections for the future include increased rates of coastal disaster (Gray, 1990), increased toxic exposures of communities (Quarantelli, 1992), and the potential for global ecological collapse with resulting mass migration and unemployment (Berger & Kelly, 1993). These and other disasters result in professionals and volunteers enacting social work roles to provide disaster relief and services. Social work roles in disaster include advocacy, psychosocial assessment, service coordination, counseling, public education, community organizing, outreach, and information and referral.

Social workers have documented or researched the profession's multifaceted involvement in a variety of types of natural and man-made disasters. Social work research in disasters includes research and intervention in natural disasters such as earthquakes (Liu, 1996; Dufka, 1988; Streeter & Gillespie, 1992), fires (Armstrong et al., 1995), hurricanes (Cherry, Cherry, & Bowie, 1995), riverine flooding (Kreuger, Stretch, & Hatfield, 1995; Sundet & Mermelstein, in this volume), and tornados (Blakeway, Bishop, & Ciaccio, 1996). As the articles in this collection show, social workers are also beginning to conduct research in technological disasters, including toxic materials and hazardous exposures (Gillespie, Rogge, & Robards, 1996; Rogge, 1995), as well as global ecological disasters (Berger & Kelly, 1993). Finally, social workers are researching collective stress situations involving mass violence (Kim-Goh, 1996; Rosenthal, 1996; Seck, 1996).

Academic Disciplines and Social Work Disaster Research

The field of disaster research is most closely associated with the academic discipline of sociology. Early studies of disaster were all conducted by sociologists, and sociologists dominated disaster research until the 1960s. The National Opinion Research Center's project on peacetime disaster in the early 1950s and the establishment of the Disaster Research Center (DRC) in 1963 promoted field research as a major method in studying disaster, and institutionalized disaster research as a field of study. Many of the earlier disaster studies in sociology were on the immediate impact phase in smaller communities. This focus soon broadened to include studies on mitigation, prevention, recovery, and reconstruction, and by the late 1960s social geographers joined sociologists in conducting disaster research (Quarantelli, 1992).

Psychology and psychiatry became actively involved in research on disasters and collective stress situations by the 1980s. Experimental psychologists, aware of the limitations in external validity of laboratory research on stress, began field research on collective stress in disaster settings. In 1980, Post-Traumatic Stress Disorder (PTSD) was formally recognized as a clinical disorder by inclusion in the third edition of the *Diagnostic and Statistical Manual of Mental Disorders* (DSM-III). Before this time it was not believed that disasters could lead to long-term stress disorders. As a result of this recognition, experimental psychologists, community psychologists, and psychiatrists began extensive research into reactions and consequences of disaster (Wilson, 1993). They likewise investigated community, social and individual mediators to these reactions, as well as formal interventions for traumatic stress disorders (Solomon, 1989).

Social work disaster research is part of this rapid worldwide expansion of disaster research in the 1980s. Just as the profession of social work borrowed knowledge first from sociology and then psychology and psychiatry, so has social work disaster research developed in the context of disaster research in sociology and psychology. Disaster research in the clinical social work has focused on the psychosocial effects of disaster on victims and workers, as well as interventions for traumatic stress disorders (Hodgkinson & Shepard, 1994; Armstrong et al., 1995; Kreuger, Stretch, & Hatfield, 1995; Siporin, 1987). This research draws primarily on research in psychology and psychiatry. The research in social work draws on psychological and psychiatric investigations of individuals' reactions to disaster, the epidemiology of traumatic stress disorders, and clinical interventions for severe reactions among victims and disaster workers (Solomon, 1989).

Social work research on disaster organizations and interorganizational coordination has primarily been based in the sociology of disasters, organizations, and interorganizational relations (Quarantelli, 1992). Disaster research in social work in this area involves research on disaster planning, preparedness, response and recovery at the organizational and interorganizational levels (Gillespie, Sherraden, Streeter, & Zakour, 1986; Smiar, 1992; Streeter & Gillespie, 1992). Research on organizations and coordination represents one of the first areas of systematic disaster research in social work, and began during the rapid expansion of disaster research in the 1980s from its origins in sociology to other disciplines and professions.

Social work research on community aspects of disaster, as the articles in this volume show, uses a systems approach and focuses on the relationships among variables at different levels of analysis. Relationships among community, interorganizational, family, and group variables are examined (Coulter & Noss, 1988; Siporin, 1987; Rogge, 1995). This area of disaster social work research, as might be expected, draws on research from a number of disciplines including psychology, sociology, and geography. Community research in both psychology and sociology is the primary foundation for this social work research area. Sociological research related to disaster, organizations, and collective behavior are also important, as is research conducted by social geographers on locational issues.

Social work disaster research in the community area is part of an effort in related disciplines to examine behavior in its broader social context (Gist & Lubin, 1989).

Two additional important areas of social work disaster research are research on disaster volunteers and minority populations. Research on volunteers in disaster has drawn heavily from sociological research on the mass assault, disaster-relevant organizations, and social support in rural community settings. Social work disaster volunteerism research focuses on the use and coordination of volunteers during disaster for social services delivery. Disaster volunteerism research in social work is a part of research on voluntary action, an interdisciplinary field with substantial involvement from sociology, political science, psychology, and anthropology.

Social work research on disaster's effects on vulnerable populations is part of the profession's mission of service to disadvantaged populations, and is based primarily on psychological studies of stress and sociological research on disasters in low-income and minority communities. Because low-income and other disadvantaged populations are often either segregated or concentrated in inner cities or rural communities (Park, 1975/1926), social geographers have also contributed to this area of social work research. This social work research is an important part of the research by psychologists and psychiatrists to understand how individual characteristics act as risk factors or mediators between trauma and stress reactions (Solomon, 1989). Social work research on minorities in disasters is also part of sociological research on increased vulnerability of various minority groups to disaster, as well as their relative lack of resources for disaster response and recovery.

Traumatic Stress Interventions

Social work interventions in disaster focus on health and mental health services to alleviate the negative emotional and health reactions which disaster survivors often experience. One avenue of current research is the investigation of the different stress responses of disaster workers, based on the prior training and certification of the service workers. As Dodds and Nuehring note, little research on the stress responses of workers has been conducted, and research on the mediating variables affecting stress reactions is needed.

Violent crime, civil unrest, and acts of terrorism and violence that affect many people represent both chronic and acute stressors, particularly for urban dwellers and inner-city residents. The Oklahoma City bombing indicates that terrorist acts can occur in any region of the United States, and violent crime has spread from inner-city areas to suburban and even rural areas. Social workers are beginning to intervene in these collective stress situations, and are using many of the same approaches used in other disaster mental health settings.

Interventions for post-traumatic stress have taken a secondary prevention approach, and have been organized into various debriefing protocols. Debriefing the victims of disaster in a timely fashion seems to prevent serious post-traumatic stress symptoms from intensifying and becoming long-term problems. Often these debriefing programs use mainstream social work groupwork methods. These promising interventions have not been carefully evaluated using adequate research designs, and should be the focus of future research in disaster (Armstrong et al., 1995). Because these interventions emphasize a strengths approach, it will be necessary to determine the effectiveness of each of the clinical interventions with specific sociodemographic client groups.

Organizational and Interorganizational Research

Social work research on networks and improved coordination will help improve response efficiency, and facilitate the growing collaboration among governmental, voluntary, and other organizations from local to federal and even international levels (Siporin, 1987; Liu, 1996). Coordination should flow downward from international disaster networks to frontline practitioners at the local level. Research in coordination can adopt a crisis intervention framework, because many of the foundations of coordination are a part of crisis intervention. Sundet and Mermelstein note that some of the foundations of coordination relevant to crisis intervention include community coalitions, mutual support, communication linkages, resource awareness and preparation, and planning for cooperative relationships.

Interorganizational relations have been shown to be causally important for disaster preparedness (Gillespie, Colignon, Banerjee,

Murty, & Rogge, 1993). Research in this area has begun to combine relational and attributional data, as well as variables at different levels of abstraction to better understand preparedness. The importance of examining variables from the micro to macro levels is a theme of the articles in this collection.

Not enough is known about the barriers and facilitators of interorganizational and program coordination (Gillespie, 1991). However, improved interorganizational relations can increase preparedness for disaster (Gillespie et al., 1993), and knowledge about coordination should be expanded to help social workers better facilitate network coordination, organizational effectiveness, and disaster preparedness. Coordination of agencies and programs can lead to benefits at the micro level, such as individual and family preparedness through increased public education. Preparedness at both micro and macro levels can improve individuals' perception of control over events, which greatly decreases psychological distress.

Volunteers

Volunteers and paraprofessionals have been widely used in disaster response both because of their availability and their presumed effectiveness in providing disaster services. Though professional disaster workers organized through a military model often resist including volunteers in disaster response, organized volunteers can improve service coordination and effectiveness of the relief effort (Zakour, in press). The relative effectiveness of volunteers versus professionals should be evaluated to determine the most appropriate complementary roles for volunteer and professional cooperation. Though the voluntary efforts of individuals is the foundation of the altruistic community and a restorative response after disaster (Barton, 1969), research on how social work professionals can bolster and increase the therapeutic community after a disaster is needed.

Risk Management for Vulnerable Populations

Further research on the vulnerability and strengths of disadvantaged populations should be conducted from a collective stress framework, as Dodds and Nuehring suggest. Low-income individuals often suffer from high levels of chronic stress, so that the added acute stress of a disaster can be overwhelming. Because individuals have varying resources and risks associated with their socioeconomic status, these strengths and risks should be assessed to provide the basis for social work interventions. An increased understanding of risks is also needed at the community level, because low-income and minority communities are also at increased risk for damage from disaster, and this damage is frequently long-lasting.

Environmental Issues

Disasters of technological and environmental origins are increasing with industrial development and ecological destruction. These disasters are often global and international in nature. They lead to severe economic, social, and cultural disruption, and are an important concern for international social work (Siporin, 1987). Perceived environmental disasters can lead to severe, long-term stress on affected communities (Coulter & Noss, 1988). According to Soliman, this stress is intensified by the anger and stigmatization which accompanies the legal struggle between victims and perpetrators of pollution and toxic contamination.

Because of social work's commitment to improving the social welfare of all people, and given its ecological perspective, there is a growing understanding of the role the profession must play in the current ecological crisis. Environmental disasters lead to economic dislocation, relocation of populations, and increased disease and mortality. Social work needs to widen its mission and ethical basis to include stewardship of environmental resources, to protect and enhance human well-being (Berger & Kelly, 1993).

Additional research on appropriate and effective roles for social workers is needed in the area of environmental disasters. Further research to determine the interactions between poverty and toxic exposures is also needed. The impact of toxic waste exposure at various levels in the social system needs to be explored in the context of community development and change. Soliman suggests that a historical perspective for research into technological disasters would be desirable. This perspective is particularly important given the longitudinal nature of chronic stress originating in toxic exposures.

Cross-Cultural and International Research

The United States is a major source of worldwide disaster assistance including international financial aid, donated materials, and other assistance from governmental and volunteer agencies based in the United States (Siporin, 1987). Given the United States' comprehensive role in disaster mitigation, preparedness, response, and recovery, social workers are involved in cross-cultural and cross-national disaster practice and research. Increased comparative research is necessary because many different cultural groups such as immigrants, people of color, and members of different nations are affected by disaster. Use of stress and person-in-environment approaches suggests that responses to disaster vary according to subculture and nationality because of differing mediating variables, including protective and risk factors. Also, the disaster efforts of social work need to be coordinated with that of other professions in many nations (Gillespie, 1991). These trends point to an increased need for comparative disaster research which is international and cross-cultural.

Improved Measurement and Theory

Improved measurement and research designs are needed to help build theories with practical applications in disaster social work. Many of the existing studies in disaster are either descriptive, or lack valid and reliable measurement as well as designs adequate for the research questions. Improved measurement and design will aid in testing conceptual models and building theories concerning social work in disasters and other traumatic stress and crisis situations important to social work (Robards, Gillespie, & Murty, 1996). Theory building is needed for understanding the different effects of disasters of differing types, duration, intensity, and predictability. An improved understanding of the effects of disasters on different levels of the social system would be one result of theory building.

Minahan and Pincus (1977) suggest that understanding and changing the patterns of linkages among various resource systems in the social environment is part of social work's mission. This suggests that theory construction in disaster research could be based on systems and path models of disasters, such as Barton's theory of collective stress (1969). Barton's collective stress and altruistic community models promote greater understanding and use of links among various resource subsystems in the emergency social system. Barton's theories contain variables at differing levels of abstraction, similar to the relationship between interorganizational collaboration and individual awareness and preparedness, as suggested by Faupel and Kartez in this volume. Barton's theory of the altruistic community is similar to the theoretical models contained herein, and it is a systems model capable of incorporating more than one level of analysis.

A further advantage of Barton's work is that it combines relational and attributional variables into a single model. This allows for a fuller understanding of disaster phenomenon (Gillespie et al., 1993). Additionally, Barton's theory allows for comparative assessments of normal or chronic conditions of stress with those of a more exceptional nature (Gillespie, 1988). Other avenues of theory could be integrated with various subsystems of Barton's theory. Crisis intervention theory offers a number of hypotheses regarding interorganizational relations, communication, community coalitions, mutual support, and awareness of and access to resources, and each of these areas is consistent with various blocks in Barton's model.

Systems conceptualizations such as Barton's might provide a basis for understanding the demands of crisis situations in relationship to the coping resources that individuals are able to marshal to meet these demands. Such models can be more completely and specifically operationalized using the relational approach of network analysis. Through systems analysis, a greater understanding of the emergency social system is possible, and use of a relational approach in disaster research emphasizes the unique contribution of social work to the field of disaster and stress research.

CONCLUSIONS

One important outcome of increased interest in disaster research in social work is the Disaster and Traumatic Stress Symposium, established in 1995 at the Annual Program Meeting (APM) of the Council on Social Work Education (CSWE). After assessing interest in a disaster symposium among social workers through an initial meeting at the APM, the present author proposed a new APM disaster symposium to the CSWE board in 1994. A sufficient number of papers submitted to the new symposium were accepted, and at the 1995 APM in San Diego three sessions with several presentations each were part of the Disaster and Traumatic Stress Symposium. Twelve papers were presented in five sessions at the CSWE meetings in 1996, and the disaster symposium is becoming institutionalized. The symposium represents an important gathering of social work disaster researchers. The Disaster and Traumatic Stress Symposium is both helping to encourage needed research in disaster social work, and highlighting the need for further research in this area.

As these articles suggest, the present status of social work disaster research indicates a number of future avenues for research. The impact of various types of disasters on victims and workers needs to be better understood, and further outcomes research on the effectiveness of various clinical treatments is needed. Additional research on the factors that facilitate coordination is needed, and this research should combine attributional and relational variables at different levels of analysis. Appropriate roles for volunteers in disaster services need to be better understood, and the effectiveness of volunteers in disaster relief should be evaluated using valid and reliable measurement instruments and experimental and quasi-experimental designs. Disadvantaged and vulnerable populations should be a focus of future social work disaster research, and the mediating protective and risk factors of special importance to each particular population need to be enumerated and understood.

The interaction of toxic exposures and poverty needs to be better understood, as does the impact of environmental disasters on different levels of the social system over historical time. Because the United States provides disaster relief on a global basis, and given the global nature of most disaster, comparative international research should be conducted with a special focus on service coordination. Social support and service coordination need to be better understood from micro to macro levels of analysis.

Improved measurement strategies would aid researchers in achieving each of the above research objectives. Theory building will be facilitated through improved measurement, and improved theory should occur through use of collective stress models such as Barton's theory of the altruistic community (1969). A stress, coping, and social support approach to disaster will both further the mission of social work, and indicate the unique value of the social work perspective for disaster research.

REFERENCES

Armstrong, K. R., Lund, P. E., McWright, L. T., & Techenor, V. (1995). Multiple stressor debriefing and the American Red Cross: The East Bay Hills Fire experience. *Social Work, 40*(1), 83-90.

Barton, A. H. (1969). *Communities in disaster: A sociological analysis of collective stress situations*. Garden City, NY: Doubleday.

Berger, R. M., & Kelly, J. J. (1993). Social work in the ecological crisis. *Social Work, 38*(5), 521-526.

Blakeway, K., Bishop, R., & Ciaccio, C. (1996, February). A descriptive study of natural helpers involved in disaster relief. In M. J. Zakour (Chair), *Disaster and Traumatic Stress Symposium*. Symposium conducted at the Annual Program Meeting of the Council on Social Work Education, Washington, DC.

Bolin, R. (1988). Response to natural disasters. In M. Lystad (Ed.), *Mental health response to mass emergencies: Theory and practice* (Brunner/Mazel Psychosocial Stress Series no. 12, pp. 22-51). New York: Brunner/Mazel.

Cherry, A. L., Cherry, M. E., & Bowie, S. L. (1995, March). Research as social action in the aftermath of Hurricane Andrew. In M. J. Zakour (Chair), *Disaster and Traumatic Stress Symposium*. Symposium conducted at the Annual Program Meeting of the Council on Social Work Education, San Diego, CA.

Coulter, M. L., & Noss, C. I. (1988). Preventive social work in perceived environmental disasters. *Health and Social Work, 13*(4), 296-300.

Dufka, C. L. (1988). The Mexico City earthquake disaster. *Social Casework, 69*(3), 162-170.

Erickson, K. T. (1976). *Everything in its path*. New York: Simon & Shuster.

Gillespie, D. F. (1988). Barton's theory of collective stress is a classic and worth testing. *International Journal of Mass Emergencies and Disasters, 6*(3), 345-361.

Gillespie, D. F. (1991). *Recommended research on coordination in the International Decade for Natural Disaster Reduction.* Unpublished manuscript,

Washington University in St. Louis, George Warren Brown School of Social Work, St. Louis, MO.

Gillespie, D. F., Colignon, R. A., Banerjee, M. M., Murty, S. A., & Rogge, M. E. (1993). *Partnerships for community preparedness* (Program on Environment and Behavior Monograph No. 54). Boulder, CO: Institute of Behavioral Science, University of Colorado.

Gillespie, D. L., Rogge, R. E., & Robards, K. J. (1996, February). Educating social workers for natural and technological disaster management. In M. J. Zakour (Chair), *Disaster and Traumatic Stress Symposium*. Symposium conducted at the Annual Program Meeting of the Council on Social Work Education, Washington, DC.

Gillespie, D. F., Sherraden, M. W., Streeter, C. L., & Zakour, M. J. (1986). *Mapping networks of organized volunteers for natural hazard preparedness* (Report no. PB87-182051/A07). Springfield, VA: National Technical Information Service.

Gist, R., & Lubin, B. (1989). Ecological and community perspectives on disaster intervention. In R. Gist & B. Lubin (Eds.), *Psychosocial aspects of disaster* (pp. 308-340). New York: Wiley & Sons.

Gray, W. M. (1990). Strong association between West African rainfall and U.S. landfall of intense hurricanes. *Science*, *249*, 1251-1256.

Hodgkinson, P. E., & Shepherd, M. A. (1994). The impact of disaster social work. *Journal of Traumatic Stress*, *7*(4), 587-600.

Kim-Goh, M. (1996, February). Psychological impact of the Los Angeles riots on Korean-American victims. In M. J. Zakour (Chair), *Disaster and Traumatic Stress Symposium*. Symposium conducted at the Annual Program Meeting of the Council on Social Work Education, Washington, DC.

Kreuger, L. W., Stretch, J. J., & Hatfield, D. (1995, September). *Assessing need for family services among flood victims*. Paper presented at the meeting of the National Association for Welfare Research and Statistics, Jackson, WY.

Liu, L. (1996, February). Government partnerships with social service agencies. In M. J. Zakour (Chair), *Disaster and Traumatic Stress Symposium*. Symposium conducted at the Annual Program Meeting of the Council on Social Work Education, Washington, DC.

Minahan, A., & Pincus, A. (1977). Conceptual framework for social work practice. In A. Minahan & S. Briar (Eds.), Conceptual Frameworks. [Special Issue]. *Social Work*, *22*(5), 347-352.

Park, R. E. (1975). The urban community as a spatial pattern and moral order. In C. Peach (Ed.), *Urban social segregation* (pp. 21-31). New York: Longman. (Original work published 1926).

Quarantelli, E. L. (1992). Disaster research. In E. Borgatta & M. Borgatta (Eds.), *Encyclopedia of sociology* (pp. 492-498). New York: Macmillan.

Robards, K. J., Gillespie, D. F., & Murty, S. A. (1996, February). Interorganizational relationships in disasters: Developing and testing a measure of coordination. In M. J. Zakour (Chair), *Disaster and Traumatic Stress Symposium*.

Symposium conducted at the Annual Program Meeting of the Council on Social Work Education, Washington, DC.

Rogge, M. E. (1995, March). Vulnerability to technological and natural hazards: Empowering community response. In M. J. Zakour (Chair), *Disaster and Traumatic Stress Symposium*. Symposium conducted at the Annual Program Meeting of the Council on Social Work Education, San Diego, CA.

Rosenthal, B. S. (1996, February). An insidious source of traumatic stress: Exposure to chronic community violence. In M. J. Zakour (Chair), *Disaster and Traumatic Stress Symposium*. Symposium conducted at the Annual Program Meeting of the Council on Social Work Education, Washington, DC.

Seck, E. T. (1996, February). Social unrest in Los Angeles: The impact of race and ethnicity. In M. J. Zakour (Chair), *Disaster and Traumatic Stress Symposium*. Symposium conducted at the Annual Program Meeting of the Council on Social Work Education, Washington, DC.

Siporin, M. (1987). Disasters and disaster aid. In A. Minahan (Ed.), *Encyclopedia of social work* (18th ed., pp. 438-449). Silver Spring, MD: National Association of Social Workers.

Smiar, N. P. (1992). Cool heads: Crisis management for administrators. *Child Welfare*, *71*(2), 147-156.

Smith, E. M., North, C. S., & Price, P. C. (1988). Response to technological accidents. In M. Lystad (Ed.), *Mental health response to mass emergencies: Theory and practice* (Brunner/Mazel Psychosocial Stress Series no. 12, pp. 52-95). New York: Brunner/Mazel.

Solomon, S. D. (1989). Research issues in assessing disaster's effects. In R. Gist & B. Lubin (Eds.), *Psychosocial aspects of disaster* (pp. 308-340). New York: Wiley & Sons.

Speizman, M. D., & Lloyd, G. A. (1965, October). School Responds to Betsy. *Postscripts: Alumni Bulletin Tulane University School of Social Work*, pp. 1-2.

Streeter, C. L., & Gillespie, D. F. (1992). Social network analysis. In D. F. Gillespie & C. Glisson (Eds.), Quantitative methods in social work: State of the art. [Special Issue]. *Journal of Social Service Research*, *16*(1/2), 201-222.

Streeter, C. L., Gillespie, D. F., Sherraden, M. W., & Zakour, M. J. (1986). Curriculum development in interorganizational coordination. *Journal of Social Work Education*, *22*(1), 32-40.

Trattner, W. (1994). *From Poor Law to welfare state* (5th ed.). New York: Free Press.

Wilson, J. P. (1993). Preface. In R. D. Allen (Ed.), Handbook of post-disaster interventions. [Special Issue]. *Journal of Social Behavior and Personality*, *8*(5), v.

Zakour, M. J. (in press). Geographic and social distance during emergencies: A path model of interorganizational links. *Social Work Research*.

A Primer for Social Work Research on Disaster

Sally Dodds
Elane Nuehring

SUMMARY. This paper offers to schools of social work a conceptual framework and specific tactics intended to position them for much-needed research roles in response to natural or technological disasters. Based on experience gained in the aftermath of Hurricane Andrew in Miami, Florida in 1992, potential research themes, needs and opportunities are identified, along with policy, organizational, and resource barriers to investigation encountered in the post-disaster context. The necessity of advance preparation for disaster research is emphasized, along with strategies for readiness. Design and methodology are discussed, and specific approaches are recommended regarding framing questions, becoming immersed in the multidisciplinary disaster services research community before the fact, research design, instrumentation, and data collection process and administration.

Based on Breznitz and Goldberger (1982), Derogatis (1982), Elliott (1982), Lazarus (1984), and Sarafino (1990), a stress-mediation theory is suggested for its capability to guide disaster-focused social work research at micro, mezzo, and macro levels.

Sally Dodds, PhD, is affiliated with University of Miami Department of Psychiatry and the Behavioral Sciences, Miami, FL. Elane Nuehring, PhD, is affiliated with Barry University School of Social Work, Miami, FL.

An earlier version of this article was presented at the 41st Annual Program Meeting of the Council on Social Work Education, San Diego, CA, March 2-5, 1995, entitled "Preparation for Disaster in Academic Settings: A Formula for Social Work Research."

[Haworth co-indexing entry note]: "A Primer for Social Work Research on Disaster." Dodds, Sally and Elane Nuehring. Co-published simultaneously in *Journal of Social Service Research* (The Haworth Press, Inc.) Vol. 22, No. 1/2, 1996, pp. 27-56; and: *Research on Social Work and Disasters* (ed: Calvin L. Streeter and Susan A. Murty) The Haworth Press, Inc., 1996, pp. 27-56. Single or multiple copies of this article are available for a fee from The Haworth Document Delivery Service [1-800-342-9678, 9:00 a.m. - 5:00 p.m. (EST). E-mail address: getinfo@haworth.com].

Pivotal research questions are posed, suggesting a disaster research agenda for social workers. Areas of inquiry best understood as *exploratory* and best approached with qualitative techniques are discussed, along with specific suggestions for the design and implementation of qualitative disaster research. Areas of inquiry best seen as *descriptive of populations and explanatory of biopsychosocial phenomena* are identified, along with recommended survey and quasi-experimental designs and recommended preparatory work to enable expedient sampling, instrumentation, and data collection. Investigation of the *effectiveness of social work interventions* in the post-disaster milieu is encouraged, along with feasible and methodologically sound quasi-experimental designs.

Measurement of critical variables and instrumentation are discussed, along with ethical issues unique to the disaster context, the necessity of effective inter-organizational and interdisciplinary collaborations, and accessing the "national and international disaster research community" for input on funding, design, and methodological conundrums that impact this fast-moving, emotionally-laden, frequently chaotic research environment. *[Article copies available for a fee from The Haworth Document Delivery Service: 1-800-342-9678. E-mail address: getinfo@haworth.com]*

INTRODUCTION

As the incidence and scale of devastation of natural and technological disasters increases (Baum, 1987; Freedy et al., 1992), schools of social work[1] need specific strategies to develop preparedness plans to conduct vital research. Although advance preparation is salient to schools situated in areas at known risk for disasters, planning is also germane to schools outside of vulnerable areas. Institutions not directly impacted by a disaster may collaborate in partnerships to support the research efforts of schools immediately affected.

This article is based on the experience of two universities in Miami (Florida) following Hurricane Andrew in 1992. The schools' roles in training, case consultation, and stress management in the post-disaster crisis intervention response led to numerous opportu-

1. While this discussion focuses on the research readiness of academic settings, there are many social work researchers in non-academic service organizations to whom these suggestions apply.

nities for social work research. However, because of barriers explained below, many such opportunities were not realized. In anticipation of future hurricane impact in this high-risk coastal region, the schools have since developed a strategy of "research preparedness." Considerations leading to this planned strategy are the focus of this article.

LESSONS IN RESEARCH PREPAREDNESS FROM HURRICANE ANDREW

In August, 1992, Hurricane Andrew left approximately 2.5 million Florida residents without electrical power, destroyed 56,000 family dwelling units, and rendered 350,000 persons homeless (CDC, 1992). The most devastating hurricane in 25 years, Andrew destroyed the entire bureaucratic infrastructure of south Dade County, requiring supplementation by the American Red Cross, the armed forces, and the Federal Emergency Management Agency (FEMA).

The Florida Department of Health and Rehabilitative Services (HRS), in collaboration with FEMA and the National Institute of Mental Health, generated a crisis response program. The core of this effort was a cadre of some 220 personnel hired to staff mobile outreach teams responsible for mental health and health assessments of survivors, crisis counseling, and referral in the post-disaster period. To support this crisis response program, the University of Miami Department of Psychiatry and the Barry University School of Social Work collaborated to provide intensive disaster-related training and support services. However, as we prepared curriculum and program activities, we were confronted by the relative scarcity of research applicable to first responders in outreach programs upon which we could base our training and support efforts.

It was further apparent that a post-disaster study population of 220 potential participants was available in the outreach teams. We were interested in measuring aspects of stress and burnout among this group, a unique sample of disaster workers in that many were themselves hurricane victims, few were licensed social workers or counselors, all were inexperienced in working out-of-doors in subtropical field conditions, and remained in the field for over a year following the storm. We also noted many other areas of potential inquiry that were (a) largely untreated in the published literature, (b) had been studied with compromised methodologies, or (c) had been investigated in the context of very different kinds of disasters, typically technological catastrophes. For example, Hurricane Andrew's impact on the unique sociodemographic region of South Florida affected many special populations and groupings that had received little or no attention in the literature with respect to the impact of disaster. These included persons with disabilities, caregivers, racial and ethnic groups, immigrants and illegal entrants, institutionalized and incarcerated groups, economically disadvantaged and homeless groups, family units, neighborhoods and communities. The long-term effects of disasters are little understood, and after a year and a half in the field, we noticed different recovery patterns among similarly situated persons. We also observed a number of subgroups who made little movement toward recovery, particularly the economically marginal. Substance abuse, family violence, and situational depression are thought to increase among disaster victims, but the correlations are not well documented in the research literature. Further, the incidence of clinically defined PTSD among disaster survivors remains in question. Nor has the literature carefully partialized the stress-producing aspects of disaster: do victims react most acutely to the actual in vivo disaster experience and the accompanying terror, to subsequent and objective losses of personal property and other tangible resources, to protracted disruption of social relationships and community services, to secondary technological accidents (spills, releases, explosions, etc.) caused by the natural disaster, or to the upheaval and frustration precipitated by the emergency assistance and insurance systems? At the organizational, interorganizational, and community levels, gaps in research coverage leave many unanswered questions salient to social work. For example, what are the barriers to and facilitating factors for effective mobilization of the emergency assistance agencies in communities of different sizes, sociocultural, and political features? How does disaster and its sequelae impact on inter-governmental and inter-organizational relationships? What are the immediate and long-term consequences of the disaster on the political, economic, demographic, social-structural and social psychological climate of communities and social networks?

Although these considerations generated many research questions for us, our own lack of preparedness hampered our investigations. Further, we observed disaster experts arrive from areas outside of our region to conduct research activities. These researchers typically employed ready-made protocols, developed during other, often non-similar, disaster events and conditions. While outside experts make essential contributions to disaster research, they lack the acumen that is possible when research is conducted by local scholars who intimately know the affected community and can access systems and structures to implement more complex designs for greater depth and sensitivity.

As local researchers, the capacity to rapidly mobilize research effectively was frustrated by a number of elements of the disaster context. In our experience, we were too impacted and too overwhelmed to locate and review appropriate literature, conceptualize meaningful questions, locate optimal instruments, devise samples, identify and obtain funding support, and conduct data collection rapidly and effectively. A pre-planned set of questions and hypotheses, variables, measures and instruments, funding mechanisms, and tentative sampling and participant selection plans were not in place. Further, only a handful of academicians in the community had pre-existing expertise in disasters; for most of us, disaster research was a new field and we needed time to learn. Particularly for academic institutions located in disaster-prone regions, this experience underscores (a) the need for advance knowledge and competency-building in disaster research, (b) advance research plans and collaborative linkages, which can be implemented readily when disaster strikes; and (c) the opportunities for meaningful disaster research at times other than proximity to an immediate disaster event.

THE STATE OF SOCIAL WORK-RELEVANT DISASTER RESEARCH

Although the disaster literature cuts across the physical, biobehavioral, and social sciences, it reflects practically no social work presence. Further, empirically based understanding of biopsychosocial phenomena surrounding disaster, at the micro, mezzo, and macro levels, is often seriously compromised as to generalizability and/or internal validity, and may be limited in coverage of populations and systems of traditional concern to social work. Consistent with these observations, in a recent comprehensive review of research on the effects of disaster on mental health, Green (1993) found only 131 quantitative, empirical studies of survivors/subjects exposed to natural or technical disaster. Of these studies, many were descriptive. The number of studies where relatively rigorous control group designs were used was less than 20%. Natural prospective (single group pre-post) designs with large numbers of subjects were few, as were natural retrospective designs with large samples. Intervention research, assessing program or treatment outcomes, was virtually non-existent, and although disaster relief systems have been the subject of considerable descriptive study (for relevant reviews, see Dynes & Tierney, 1994; Quarantelli, 1987, 1990; 1992), evaluative research informing disaster response service systems and structures continues to need significant development (Green, in press). In social work, research on disasters is only now beginning to emerge (examples include the work of Ager & Zakour, 1995; Cherry & Cherry, 1995; Gillespie et al., 1986; Rogge, 1995). Further, there has been little systematic dissemination of information about disasters and disaster response to social workers through the established journals, conferences, and other communication channels of the profession.

Thus, many areas of potential inquiry clearly remain at all levels of study: exploratory, descriptive, epidemiological, explanatory, and evaluative of intervention and program outcomes. Accordingly, designs are in order that emphasize qualitative methods, surveys, especially those with longitudinal components, field experiments, and quasi-experiments, commensurate with the research purposes. Myers (1991) calls for rigorous research that reaches the field in understandable, applicable terms on the differential effects of various forms of disaster. These include, among many others: disaster sequelae such as substance abuse, domestic violence, depression and suicide; incidence of verifiable PTSD; the effects of disaster on special populations such as the aged, single parents, persons with disabilities, and various ethnic and cultural groups, elders; effects of the "second disaster" created by the complex disaster recovery, construction, and insurance bureaucracy; anniversary reactions; and, effects of interventions such as debriefing and support groups. Additionally, research that attends to the special risks, needs, and coping of disaster response personnel, especially those who are also disaster survivors, is notably scarce (Green, 1993).

However, if expedient execution of studies is to occur, a research template, consistent with federal policy toward disaster victims, needs to be in place before the disaster strikes. When no specific disaster is imminent, or when public and professional focus on a recent disaster event recedes, the opportunity must be seized to plan and fund studies appropriate for future disaster events and to execute the innumerable disaster-relevant studies that can be accomplished outside of a specific disaster experience. The following sections of this article will highlight selected conceptual, design, and implementation considerations to facilitate much-needed disaster research. While an exhaustive examination of the possibilities for study is beyond the scope of this paper, the intent is to entice social work scholars to germinate a research response to disaster that is capable of informing professional practice and education.

A RESEARCH PRIMER FOR SOCIAL WORK RESEARCH IN DISASTERS

Conceptual Models

In designing empirical disaster research, it is critical to begin with a clearly conceptual model capable of delineating the potential variables to be investigated, as well as their potential inter-relationships. The applied use of such models can partially alleviate the diverse findings related to disaster effects. Arguably, the most useful models for disaster research are based on a stress construct, and examine the relationship between the disaster as a stressor event and its subsequent outcomes on affected persons and systems. Stress models are extremely appropriate paradigms for social work research in disasters, for they can be broadened to include micro, mezzo, and macro level variables, place emphasis on the person-environment fit, support adaptation rather than pathology, and suggest practice applications for individuals, families, small groups, organizations, and communities.

At their most basic stimulus-response (S-R) formulation, stressors are typically seen as external events or conditions originating in both the physical and social environment that impose on target systems. Several properties of stress stimuli may be applied to disaster research which affect the impact on the individual or collectivity, either quantitatively or qualitatively. One category of properties is organized around the *duration of the stressor* (for example, acute, time-limited stressors; stressor sequences over time as the result of an initiating event; chronic, intermittent stressors that may occur once a day, once a week, once a month) (Elliott and Eisdorfer, 1982). Another property is the *demand of the stressor* (that is, types and magnitude of adjustments required, extent of controllability, increased or diminished burden due to the capacity of the stressor to unite or react with other stressors) (Lazarus, 1984). Still other aspects of disaster as a stimulus consider the *type of event*. Types of disasters include natural events vs. technological or human precipitated accidents, as well as human directed events growing out of mass conflict (such as war or civil disturbance). Finally, the defined *scope of impact*, whether community-wide or affecting limited collectivities, is central to characterizing the disaster as a stressor event.

The response side of the S-R equation focuses on reactions to stressors by the individual, group, organization, community, or other affected system. For individuals, stress responses have two interrelated components which have implications for disaster research. Psychological response involves the subjective, phenomenological experience of stress. This subjectivity leads to behaviors and thought patterns that are classified as the effects of stress (for example, the expression of emotion, performance deterioration, or symptom manifestation) (Sarafino, 1990). The second component, physiological response, involves heightened bodily arousal and health-related outcomes. Extending the stress model to collectivities, the social-psychological climate and functioning of families (nuclear and extended), neighborhoods, organizations, and interorganizational networks are influenced by disaster stimuli, and social pattern disruption occurs at all social and organizational levels.

Simple stimulus-response models of stress are restrained from considering important mediating variables, and other definitions of stress have evolved to consider this missing dimension. A second approach to defining stress describes it as a process that includes stressors and responses, but adds the dimension of the relationship between the individual and the environment (Lazarus, 1984). A collectivity may also be considered in relationship to its environment. The target system, then, is an active agent capable of influencing the impact of the stressor through behavioral, cognitive, emotional, organizational, and social strategies referred to as protective factors if they buffer the target system from adverse responses and risk factors if they heighten the target system's vulnerability to adverse responses.

Two approaches to relational definitions of stress are important to social work research in disasters. The first, an interactional point of view, emphasizes trait characteristics of the individual or other system, which act as major mediating mechanisms between stimulus characteristics of the environment and the responses they invoke (Derogatis, 1982). Because of its emphasis on unidirectional causality, this approach views the target system as reactive. The second relational approach is transactional: not only does the individual or collectivity mediate the effect of environmental stimuli in a linear manner, but also the continuous interactions between the characteristics of the responding system can affect and become a significant part of the environment (Derogatis, 1982). Transactional stress theorists view responding systems as active and dynamic, and use a systems approach to stress models with feedback loops that allow for constant interplay among the components of the system to provide equilibrium (Derogatis, 1982).

Relational definitions of stress that highlight the importance of individual and group differences provide important research dimensions that are necessary to complement S-R variables. First, because collectivities have characteristics of their own, research can include the systematic exposure of different populations, social groups, organizations, and institutions to a specific stressor (or disaster event) (Goldberger and Breznitz, 1982). Second, the impact of a given stressor on different individuals or units within the same group of units gives rise to the study of individual differences to stressors (Goldberger & Breznitz, 1982). Among the individual and group differences of most relevance are those that concern the perception and cognitive appraisal of stressors on the part of individuals, and social definitions, belief systems, and structural properties at collective levels. In turn, these variables play a major role in the coping or other adaptive transactions between the systems and the stressors (Goldberger & Breznitz, 1982). Third, emphasis on within-group differences provides the opportunity to investigate a range of outcomes that results from stress. These include minor changes in individual, group, and organizational behavior, dramatic psychological and physical clinical conditions among individuals (Goldberger & Breznitz, 1982), and major alterations in collective structures and functions and institutional arrangements.

It must be noted that research using transactional definitions often proves difficult. The keystone construct of transactional definitions (that is, relevant mediating mechanisms constantly affecting, and being affected by, the demand characteristics of the environment), creates problems in measurement. The dynamic reciprocal relationship constantly alters the values of the components, demanding careful sequential measurement approaches (Derogatis, 1982). However, both approaches are necessary, and investigators should focus on mechanisms of interactions to better understand the variables and the functional relationships between antecedent conditions and subsequent outcomes.

Because of the many definitions of stress that have been developed to meet specific needs for different types of research, an overarching conceptual framework into which all definitions of stress research seems to fit was developed by the Institute of Medicine (Elliott and Eisdorfer, 1982) (see Figure 1), and is exceptionally suited to social work research in disasters. This Framework for Stress Research is as follows: The stress response can be divided into four fundamental elements–activators (x), reactions (y), consequences (z), and mediators. Activators (or stressors) are defined as potential events or conditions in the environment that change the present state of an individual or collective. An activator does not need to be an actual stimulus, because even the absence (or threat)

FIGURE 1. Framework for Stress Research

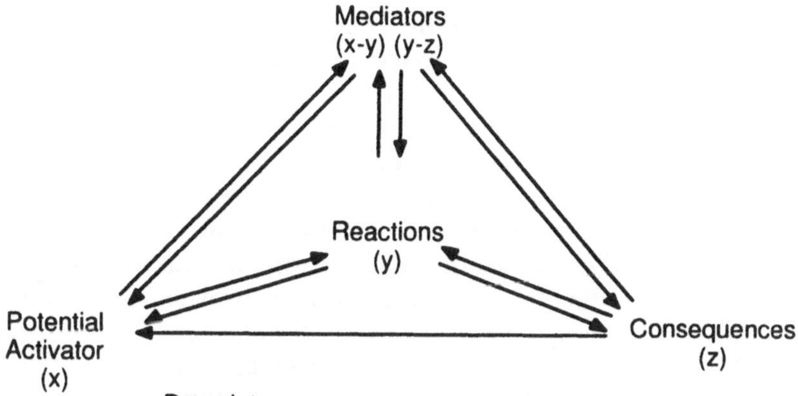

Descriptors:
Organizational Level
Intensity
Quantity
Temporal Pattern
Evaluative Quality (for Consequences only)

of an event may be important. Activators may be described in terms of their intensity, quantity, and pattern in time. Furthermore, activators may act at any level of the organization (Elliott and Eisdorfer, 1982). This is analogous to conceptualizing systems in micro, mezzo, and macro levels.

Activators elicit reactions. Reactions are biological, behavioral, psychological, or social responses of an individual or collective system to a stressor and, like activators, may occur at many different levels of organizational complexity. They may also be described in terms of their intensity, quantity, and temporal pattern.

Consequences are viewed as physical, behavioral, psychological, or social results of such reactions. Because distinctions between reactions and consequences are not always easy to make, the terms are used to differentiate between transient responses to specific activators (reactions) and more prolonged and/or cumulative effects of those reactions (consequences). Consequences could be any result of a system's reactions to the disaster. Individuals may experience changes in psychological states (e.g., depression, anxiety);

changes in social roles or status (e.g., homelessness, unemployment); changes in behavior (e.g., substance use, domestic violence); or changes in health conditions (e.g., heart attack). Families and defined groups such as civic associations or residential blocks may experience intensified interaction and affiliation as members share their circumstances or join in altruistic efforts. Organizations may see plunges in efficiency and staff morale as employees who are disaster victims cope with recovery demands. New policies and procedures may emerge. Organizations may re-locate, or may be abolished. At the community and interorganizational levels, new coalitions, coordinating mechanisms, and disaster response plans may evolve. Consequences thus can occur at all levels of organizational complexity, and also may differ from one another in intensity, quantity, and temporal pattern. Importantly, a consequence also has an evaluative component relative to some collective or personal standard. It may be considered bad (e.g., ill health), good (e.g., neighborhood cohesiveness), or neutral. For these reasons, "evaluative assessments must be limited to consequences, rather than to either the responsible stressor or the intervening reaction" (Elliott and Eisdorfer, 1982, p. 22).

Mediators are intervening filters that act on each stage of the sequence to produce variations in the x-y-z sequence. In addition to mediating effects, intervening variables in stress research are described as having direct, moderating, or buffering effects, and differentiation among them should be made clear. Many processes filter activators in the x-y step to reactions. At the micro level of individuals, biological variables (such as genetic make-up or the presence of biologically-based psychiatric disorders), psychological variables (such as strong denial or history of traumatic experiences), social variables (such as role or class), and physical variables (such as crowded housing conditions) may substantially alter the significance of a specific potential activator. At the mezzo levels of families or small, defined groups, numerous variables may influence the impact of an activator. Among these are structure and composition, social roles and role functioning, communication, control and decision-making, coping methods, cohesiveness, and types and extent of social support. At the macro level of large organizations and institutions, mediators of disaster effects may include, for example, disruption of the demand and supply for products and services and degree of bureaucratization. The impact of activators within interorganizational networks may be filtered by the system's history of collaboration and cooperation (frequency and intensity), the system's sheer size and complexity, and its formalization. Effects of activators on whole communities may be buffered by geographic features, the nature and strength of the local economy, the effectiveness of leadership, political participation and power relationships, and characteristics of the post-disaster environment such as duration of disruption, resources to aid recovery, nature of media coverage, and the effectiveness of the relief bureaucracy in providing expeditious, coordinated, accessible, and non-chaotic assistance.

Disaster Phases and Research Implementation

Disasters have been conceptualized as progressing through several phases: the interim or mitigation phase during which no specified disaster is imminent; the immediate pre-disaster preparation phase when an identified disaster is anticipated and the period of direct disaster impact; the immediate post-disaster rescue and relief phase; and the prolonged recovery and re-building phase (American Red Cross, 1993). Two of these phases are proximate to the event: the time of immediate anticipation of, and preparation for, a predicted, imminent, and specific event; and the immediate rescue and relief effort following impact. The recovery and rebuilding phase may occur over weeks, months, or years–as long as the disaster aftermath persists as an observable theme in the affected community. The interim or mitigation phase also may endure briefly or for years. Each of the disaster phases lends itself differentially to research themes at all system levels. Table 1 suggests a variety of sample research questions and study approaches consistent with the demands of given disaster stages. However, it is the interim or mitigation phase where essential planning must occur in addition to an active research agenda.

Research Planning During the Interim or Mitigation Phase

During times when no specific disaster is the focus of recovery efforts and no specific event is known to be approaching, anticipa-

TABLE 1. The Phases of Disaster and Examples of Disaster Research Questions

Phases of Disaster: Interim or Mitigation	*Possible Designs, Subjects, Sampling*	*Measurement & Data Collection Approaches*	*Analysis Strategy*
Micro: To what extent do disaster anniversary dates, annual occurrences of high risk seasons, and other disaster reminders evoke *responses* among survivors? What responses? For how many years after a disaster? Are some groups more likely than others to be adversely affected by disaster recollections: those whose lives were in grave peril or who lost significant others in the disaster, children, persons with various disabilities, persons with fewer lifetime disaster exposures, and the like?	1. Follow-up of panels of subjects included in studies implemented in the immediate relief and prolonged recovery phases; self-administered mail questionnaires or telephone interviews. 2. Telephone survey screening for survivors, retrospectively establishing exposure, and assessing current cognitive and emotional involvement with the disaster, including the effects of anniversaries.	Objective behavior report items and measures of frequency of thinking and talking about the disaster and the intensity of emotion connected with thoughts of the disaster; disaster exposure assessment items as needed.	Regression & logistic regression
Mezzo: Can mental health professionals specifically *trained* for disaster response be differentiated from untrained professionals in response to simulated disaster emergency situations, controlling for disaster mental health experience, credentials, and total professional practice experience?	Simulation experiment comparing crisis response and personal coping strategies among a group of LCSWs trained in the APA-Red Cross Disaster Mental Health Certification Program, with a group of uncertified LCSWs, matched on professional experience and disaster-specific experience.	Standardized measures of personal problem-solving or coping; original items tapping crisis and disaster knowledge and beliefs and self-perceived response to a disaster situation.	MANOVA
Macro: What is the differential vulnerability of neighborhoods and communities to the effects of technological disasters, including secondary technological disasters (spills, releases, explosions, etc.) caused by natural disasters? What are the characteristics of areas that *mediate risk*? Are there social action implications for areas at high risk?	Identification of neighborhood areas (e.g., census tracts, voting precincts, elementary school divisions, blocks) or community units, determination of their proximity to technological sites, the relative vulnerability of such installations to both primary technological and natural disaster-caused mishaps, the level of protection in place, the added disaster preparedness measures necessary in light of the prospects of technological disasters including those secondary to natural disaster. Assessment of neighborhood/community awareness of the potential for primary and secondary technological disasters and of community/neighborhood capacity for organized social action to mitigate technological hazards.	Analysis of archival information on areas, their sociodemographic attributes, industrial/technological data. Focused interviews re: natural disaster damage mitigation measures in place. Standardized community surveys re: awareness and action capacity.	Identification of patterns & descriptive/subgroup analysis. Data could be designed to lend themselves to structural equation modeling; log-linear techniques may also be usable.

Phases of Disaster: Imminent Pre-Disaster	*Possible Designs, Subjects, Sampling*	*Measurement Approaches*	*Analysis Strategy*
Micro: Do social service and mental health personnel vary in individual *reaction* to pending disaster, and related priority setting commitments, behavioral, psychological, emotional, and role-functioning *consequences* according to *mediators* such as their ethno-cultural background? their previous disaster experiences? their training? their position in the agency?	One-shot survey of probability samples of agency staffs via short self-completed group-administered questionnaires or structured, brief interviews.	Objective items measuring individual characteristics, background, organizational role/position; scales designed to tap behavioral, cognitive, emotional, and role-functioning dimensions of interest.	Descriptive-comparative subgroup analyses; ANOVA, MANOVA if data can meet assumptions.
Mezzo: What levels of disaster preparation, evacuation and sheltering support & assistance are understood by families to be available to them, and from what formal & informal sources? Does knowledge of and perceived access to assistance resources vary according to sociodemographic attributes of families and neighborhoods? Does level of perceived support and assistance *mediate* apprehension and stress levels in families?	Door-to-door survey of random samples of households, with census tracts (or blocks) randomly chosen from strata grouped reflect SES and ethnic contrasts.	Objective items measuring formal and informal sources of support and assistance families believe to be available to them to protect their property and ensure their safety.	Descriptive-comparative subgroup analyses; loglinear analysis or logistic regression, depending on level of measure of defined dependent variables.
Macro: At the organizational level of *reponse to pending disaster*, what provisions are in place for disabled patients/residents in out-of-home care facilities (hospitals, residential treatment programs, group homes, etc.) in the public, private, non-profit, and for-profit sectors in the event of an evacuation order? in the event of prolonged service disruption?	Telephone survey; in large communities, random samples of facilities based on stratification by organizational form and disability group served; in small communities, the population of facilities.	Objective questions specifying emergency provisions, numbers of clients involved.	Descriptive-comparative subgroup analyses; loglinear analysis or logistic regression, depending on level of measure of defined dependent variables.

TABLE 1. (continued)

Phases of Disaster: Immediate Relief & Rescue	*Possible Designs, Subjects, Sampling*	*Measurement & Data Collection Approaches*	*Analysis Strategy*
Micro: What types of psychological and physical *stressors* impact disaster relief workers in the short (and long) run post disaster? What are the respective *durations and demands* of the identified stressors? How do individuals *react*? What are the longer-term *consequences* for performance and psychological symptomatology? Do traits (e.g., coping styles) and/or circumstances (e.g., personal level of exposure to the disaster's effects) of individuals mediate reactions and consequences?	1. Field experiment; subjects exposed, comparison group unexposed; post-test only. OR. . . 2. Natural prospective; multiple point baseline data collected on subjects (single group) before and periodically after exposure to disaster.	Standardized measures of personal & job stress, situational depression, anxiety, and mediators such as social support, coping style; disaster exposure/loss of resources assessment	MANOVA for multiple dependent variable models with multiple factors and covariates; discriminant analysis
Mezzo: At the work unit/team level, what *mediates* disaster relief staff performance and morale more effectively: a program of cognitive stress inoculation & reduction or a program of physical recreation & exercise?	1. Experiment: randomly assigned subjects in respective treatment conditions compared; pre-intervention and post-intervention testing, or post-testing only. OR. . . 2. Quasi-experiment; non-equivalent non-randomized subjects in respective treatment conditions compared; pre- and post-testing.	Agency performance data or self-evaluation of performance; standardized measures of job stress & morale.	ANOVA models
Macro: At the organizational level of *reaction & consequences*, what degree of organizational disablement and incapacity occurs in social & mental health services in the immediate post-disaster situation? What functions are disrupted? For how long? What functions continue? What efforts are made for clients who are victims? What allowances are made for staff who are also victims? What effects are seen in employee turnover, absenteeism, client withdrawal from services?	Key informant interviews with agency heads, supervisors; review of program documents and contracts for service; focused interviews with workers. Conduct interviews and documents analysis within first 2 months, repeat at 6-7 months and 1+ year.	Focused and/or structured-open-ended interviews; documents content analysis.	Identification of patterns in traits and properties; classification & generation of typologies

Phases of Disaster: Prolonged Recovery & Re-Building	*Possible Designs, Subjects, Sampling*	*Measurement Approaches*	*Analysis Strategy*
Micro: Do support groups at churches, the workplace, or other settings assist disaster survivors in the reduction of their perceived stress and psychological symptomatology as the struggle of rebuilding takes place?	1. Experiment; treated subjects compared with untreated or alternatively treated equivalent control group; pre- and post-testing, or post-testing only. 2. Quasi-experiment; treated subjects compared with untreated or alternatively treated non-equivalent control group; pre- and post-testing. 3. Single treatment group, repeated measures/ multiple point baseline.	Standardized measures of stress, situational depression, anxiety, and for the quasi-experimental or single group repeated measures models, mediators such as social support, coping style.	MANOVA
Mezzo: What *mediating* attributes and experiences characterize the subset of families who are delayed in their recovery and re-building efforts, and what *consequences* does protracted delay in recovery have on their stress and functioning?	Identification of purposive sample of "still struggling" families at a point when the majority of impacted families have recovered; identify an SES-matched group of families whose recovery is judged complete.	Standardized measures of family stress and coping; objective sociodemographic measures; items tapping disaster exposure & losses, confounding events, "second disaster" phenomena	Discriminant analysis
Macro: What is the *impact of disaster and post-disaster recovery efforts* on low income housing stock and on chronic homelessness?	Natural prospective; multiple point baseline and post-disaster data collected from housing authority and county assessor's records documenting low income housing resources before and after; supplemented by counts of homeless individuals and families (ideally pre-disaster counts will exist for comparison).	Archival data analysis; censuses of homeless persons	Regression

1. Data collected in the immediate disaster aftermath may be the basis for a repeated measures follow-up plan extending into the long-run recovery phase.

2. A general rule of thumb to guide the choice of numbers of subjects in experimental groups is as follows: Assuming directional hypotheses and one-tailed tests of significance at pr = .05 will be used (or a two-tailed test at pr = .10), and further assuming that 80% power is acceptable, about 175 subjects per group will be needed to detect relatively weak effects of .25; to detect moderate effects of .40, 65 subjects per group will be needed; to detect large effects, say .80, 20 subjects per group will be sufficient. For a full discussion of the interplay among significance, power, effect size and needed sample size, see Lipsey (1990).

3. Accepted methods of counting and estimating homeless persons are discussed in Appelbaum (1990).

tory mitigation efforts can occur in the interests of minimizing the effects of future disasters, at the time they occur. Typically, individual and collective activities focus on review of prior disaster events and planning and preparedness strategies for future events. This rule is no less salient for social work researchers to conduct vital preparatory activities for disaster event investigations and to implement research that lends itself to the interim period.

Critical to efficient implementation of research in the immediate pre- and post-disaster phases is development of interorganizational collaborations well in advance of a disaster event. Two possible post-disaster scenarios should be considered in pre-planning these collaborative relationships. One potential circumstance is that the school (or other organization) and substantial numbers of its personnel are spared significant damage. In this situation, although the research organization can itself launch a planned investigation, it is necessary to have had prior understandings forged with local human service and emergency assistance agencies to the degree that their help is needed to identify participants or other aspects of data collection. The second conceivable situation is that the school or organization and its personnel have sustained serious disaster damage. In this event, planned local collaborations are still central, but additional advance collaborative arrangements with near-by sister schools or other research-capable organizations can allow the data collection and processing to proceed in a timely manner.

Although not all research relies upon inter-organizational cooperation (for example, sample surveys of the general public), such collaborations can foster an atmosphere of good will toward the research activities that may be difficult to achieve in the competing priorities of preparing for an imminent event and in the chaotic post-disaster environment. Social work researchers should consider several potential partner systems for collaboration, including local emergency management authorities, local service delivery agencies, other local academic institutions, and schools and organizations located away from the disaster region. With advance planning, research questions can be designed to inform critical aspects of the disaster response, from evacuation and emergency sheltering and relief to the extended recovery operation. Arrangements can be made to access populations through response system operations.

Questions about research ethics and funding support can be considered outside of a crisis context. Advance agency-academic agreements to permit faculty and graduate students to implement research in the agency context may be addressed. Provisions for client privacy, and mechanisms for informed consent can be put into place, particularly when the data to be collected is in a clinical context. Structures can be identified for data processing and analysis at alternative sites if computer facilities are out of order. Discussions and collaborations may be formalized in advance through letters of agreement or contractual arrangements. Importantly, collaborations should have sufficient flexibility to allow all collaborators to respond to unforeseen problems and conditions created by the disaster. In addition to pre-arranged collaborations, successfully implemented disaster research requires technical readiness.

Qualitative and quantitative designs can be pre-planned, with advance preparation directed toward framing and focusing the study, assembling and reviewing related literature (and maintaining currency in the literature archive), and determining the unit(s) of observation (e.g., perceptions, behaviors, processes, events). Data collection strategies can be selected in advance, and the necessary supplies assembled for field observation, in-depth interviews, self-administered and telephone surveys, focus groups, review of documents, films, videos, or photographs, or use of unobtrusive measures. Importantly, it is necessary to have alternative versions of instruments suitable for a back-up data collection approach in the event that the disaster makes the original strategy unfeasible. For example, if telephone service proves to be unreliable or unavailable in the impact area, methods for field interviewing should be queued for implementation. To the degree possible, the accessing, sampling, recruiting, and securing the informed consent of participants should be in place, with needed organizational arrangements anticipated, discussed, and documented among cooperating entities. For example, if the investigation will rely on observation and in-depth interviewing in public shelters, a tentative research plan should be negotiated in advance, a pre-approved proposal maintained on file, and ongoing understandings with the local emergency assistance program reviewed and updated. Importantly, ethical concerns such as the protection of disaster victims from added stress induced by a data collection process should be addressed. A written proposal will be needed to comply with Institutional Review Board (IRB) processes found in most academic and other research settings, and it can serve as an advance step toward funding the research.

Much needed in disaster research are longitudinal studies of panels and cohorts. However, these designs require additional pre-planning to conduct follow-up of specific individuals, families, groups, organizations or communities in panel studies and to implement subsequent sampling and data collection for cohort approaches. Again, interorganizational relationships need to be in place if they are to serve as the necessary access-points to units of study.

When explanation of biopsychosocial, social group, organizational, and community phenomena is the research aim, survey designs with sample sizes large enough to support multivariate analyses are important. However, the strongest explanatory designs are those that approach experimental control to the greatest degree possible by simulating the manipulation of the independent variable (that is, the disaster) by comparing victims with a carefully chosen, unexposed comparison group or groups. For purposes of studying the impact of the disaster on individuals, one of the strongest quasi-experimental designs feasible is likely to be the comparison group, post-only study (Green, 1993). This demands, in addition to general design and instrumentation, anticipation of options likely to be available for recruitment of appropriate control groups. Depending upon the predictability of the disaster (e.g., volcano eruptions, hurricane season, etc.), advance arrangements can be formulated with partner institutions, which are less at risk for the disaster's impact, to collect comparison group data.

While advance planning for non-equivalent comparison groups enhances the probability of sound comparison and contrast, the absence of true equivalent control necessarily threatens the internal validity of studies of disaster effects and, similarly, of disaster service effectiveness based on treated and untreated or differently treated comparison groups. However, measures can be taken in the choice of comparison groups that will allay, to some extent, the obvious limitations of non-equivalent comparisons.

1. Researchers should strive to identify comparison groups of the same size in comparable settings and situations, untouched by the given disaster (or other recent catastrophic events), and control for known correlates of trauma and disaster response. For example, in a study of mental health professionals and compassion fatigue, as many as possible of the extraneous variables of potential importance in predicting the dependent variable should be controlled. For example, licensed social workers without prior disaster experience in structurally similar mental health centers in similar communities unaffected by the disaster should be compared. In a study of disaster coping among caregivers, persons of the same age range, gender and ethnicity caring for the same category of persons (for example, an aged parent, mentally ill adult child, significant other with AIDS) should be compared. In a study of post-disaster organizational climate and commitment, organizations of like structure, function, size, complexity, formalization, centralization, and auspices should be the units of analysis.
2. It may be possible to match participant-for-participant on critical characteristics. For example, in a study of post-disaster stress among municipal police officers, a collaborating police department in a pre-chosen comparison community can be supplied with profiles of needed participants (for example, one female, 32 years old, single, six years of police experience) with the request that a "close" match be recruited.
3. Conditions permitting, it may be justifiable to invest in pre-disaster pre-testing, which will allow for identification and control of pre-exposure group differences. For example, in a high-frequency environment such as the Mississippi floodplain, the east coast of Florida, or the geologic fault lines of California, baseline data on consumers of clubhouse model psychosocial rehabilitation programs in half a dozen communities could supply the necessary baseline to rule out, or rule in, pre-exposure group differences.

Another quasi-experimental design involves repeated measures using single groups of participants with numbers of baseline measures adequate to detect post-disaster change. In the case of repeated measures designs, or even with single-group pre-post designs with one pre-test (useful given large enough numbers of participants to achieve statistical power), the foresighted researcher needs to determine how to obtain baseline measures for persons at risk to be victims of disaster. In some cases, pre-measures may be available as part of non-disaster-related research in progress, actuarial and health care utilization data, epidemiological data, or needs assessment studies. If research can be designed to access and involve certain clinical populations, baseline data may be available as part of existing biopsychosocial assessments maintained in clinical records and/or clinic information systems. Similar to longitudinal surveys, if multiple post-test repeated measures designs are attempted, systems for maintaining contact with participants need to be devised. Needless to say, a post-disaster context is not a smoothly managed laboratory, and the field experiments that are possible engender justifiable criticism around threats to internal validity.

Intervention research, aimed at the effectiveness of disaster response programs and interventions, is sorely needed and requires similar anticipatory strategy. Quasi-experimental and experimental designs, utilizing control and comparison groups, along with pre- and post-tests, or single group repeated measures designs can be formulated in advance, with measurement instruments, participant selection procedures, and potential service provider settings, predetermined. Likewise, in the interests of assessing treatment outcomes, single system designs can be devised, along with strategies for putting them in place in provider agencies.

Program and practice evaluations, similar to field experiments with clinical populations, which require provider involvement and a commitment of agency resources, may be impractical in the aftermath of disaster. Hence, academic institutions should expect to furnish, via faculty and students, the necessary personnel to implement efforts. Of course, agency-academic agreements and client permissions necessary to permit faculty and students to implement evaluation research in the agency context should be addressed beforehand.

Measurement Considerations

In quantitative studies, at micro, mezzo, and macro levels, choice of variables and units of analysis will vary. However, measurement and instrumentation will generally involve: (a) self-administered survey questionnaires or interview protocols designed to elicit "objective" information about the respondent's circumstances, characteristics, behaviors, and experiences; (b) psychometric scales designed to indirectly tap subjective states such as emotions, attitudes, orientations, and beliefs, or multidimensional, complex patterns of behavior or styles; and (c) rating protocols or tallying systems for use by observers, informants, or content analysts. Often, an instrument will include aspects of both objective and subjective measurement. In qualitative studies at all systems levels, interview protocols, observational protocols, audio and video recorders will be deployed.

Whether the approach is qualitative, quantitative, or a combination, generating and organizing survey items is also necessary advance work. Disaster exposure is intricate to capture and measure. Among others, for individuals, families, and some small group units of study, it involves issues such as proximity to the disaster, physical injury, psychological shock, loss of material and intangible resources, social support system upheaval, relocation, and exposure to the death, injury, and losses of others. The disaster experience will differ according to its impact sphere: whole geopolitical communities or circumscribed segments of the community or population, as is usually the case with transportation catastrophes, some technological accidents such as explosions, and mass killings. It will also vary according to the type of disaster: natural, such as hurricanes, earthquakes, volcanic eruptions, floods; technological, such as oil spills, airline crashes, explosions, and massive contaminations; or conflict-precipitated wars, riots, and acts of terrorism. Researchers are urged to obtain and study survey instruments used in other disaster research, obtain indicated permissions to use and/or modify such instruments, and prepare a field-ready survey protocol to keep on the shelf, ideally in sufficient numbers to at least begin to query the pre-designed sample of respondents expeditiously. Attention must also be given to multiple-language versions and cultural sensitivity as indicated.

With respect to psychometric scales, in many cases the constructs likely to be of interest in studying disaster impact at the micro level are measurable with published, validated tests of stress, coping, anxiety, depression, and the like. Researchers can identify promising tests, establish their availability (and costs if they are commercially published), and attend to the needs for language translations and age-appropriate versions for the target participants.

If survey data are to be collected by telephone, scales with more than five or six items may prove unfeasible. Telephone survey researchers should therefore choose brief scales or settle for subscales of longer instruments in order to realistically measure subjective constructs with telephone technology. If telephone surveying is to be used, instruments should be set up in a format suitable for telephone surveyors to use with minimum practice.

Finally, advance instrument preparation should include a complete pre-test process. Regardless of the thoroughness of advance groundwork, in an actual disaster situation, there will always be the need to make some changes based on unanticipated exigencies. The goal of advance readiness is to have in place a plan and procedures that are as field-ready as possible. Anything that can be done ahead should be done ahead, because the disaster context will provide many unforeseen issues that will require methodological and strategic attention.

Funding

Determining sources of disaster research funding also requires advance groundwork. Several mechanisms for such support exist. Importantly, the National Institute of Mental Health (NIMH), through its RAPID grants program (Rapid Assessment Post-Impact of Disaster) quickly disseminates research funding to a level of $50,000 for direct costs. Issued through Program Announcement PA-91-04 by the Traumatic Stress Research Program of the Violence and Traumatic Stress Research Branch of the NIMH, this mechanism requires eligible applicants to complete an abbreviated version of the standard USPHS-398 application kit. These applications may be submitted at any time and will receive expedited review, based on criteria that require forethought: clearly discernible research design, involving generation and/or testing of hypotheses; rationale for the proposed methodology; feasibility of the proposed research; relation of the project to future plans; availability of adequate facilities and resources necessary for the research; appropriateness of budget estimates for the proposed research activities; qualifications of the research personnel; adequacy of provisions for the protection of human subjects.

Within the context of their standard quarterly review cycle, the Traumatic Stress Research Program will also consider full proposals related to the mental health consequences of disaster, mediating factors apparent in disaster reactions, and related research. Recipients of "RAPID" grants may use this standard mechanism to extend the amount or time frame of an award.

Outside of the NIMH, other arms of the NIH with potential interest in disaster-related research include the National Institute on Drug Abuse (NIDA) and the National Institute on Alcohol and Alcoholism (NIAAA) if a focus on substance abuse as a disaster sequela are developed. Within the Substance Abuse and Mental Health Services Agency (SAMHSA), the research agenda is largely concerned with intervention effectiveness. Researchers are advised to prepare brief concept papers and ask for the reaction of staff members at the most appropriate center within SAMHSA: the Center for Mental Health Services, the Center for Substance Abuse Prevention, or the Center for Substance Abuse Treatment.

Other sources for advance inquiry as to the availability for research support include the National Science Foundation and the Veterans Administration. The Natural Hazards Research and Applications Information Center in Boulder, Colorado, issues an annual request for proposals and makes available Quick Response Grants in amounts up to $3,000 to researchers prepared to mount an investigation in a disaster situation in the predictable future. Advance investigation of research support should also be made of foundations and philanthropic organizations.

The Ethics of Disaster Research

Research ethics and sensitivity to disaster victims' situations requires thoughtful planning to ensure that research efforts do not confound recovery efforts or add to individuals' distress. Ethical research with human subjects rests on the three principles of beneficence, respect, and justice. That is, the research must maximize valuable outcomes for science, society, and the individual subject while minimizing risk or harm; the individual subject's autonomy and self-determination must be safeguarded; and reasonable, nonexploitive procedures must be administered fairly and considerately (Sieber, 1992). These principles are operationalized by the federal government in the Belmont Report (National Commission for Protection of Human Subjects of Biomedical and Behavioral Research, 1978) and the Code of Federal Regulations (45 CFR 46) pursuant to the National Research Act (PL 93-348). Additionally, most colleges, universities, and many other organizations with research components have established an Institutional Review Board consistent with the National Research Act that elaborates the given institution's policies around research participant safety. Protections assured under this framework, guided by the Belmont Report, emphasize a participant's privacy (ensured through anonymity or confidentiality provisions) and right to grant informed consent to participate in research. Informed consent presumes that sufficient information is given for a competent potential participant (or a legal guardian) to decide her or his willingness, and that consent be sought without coercion of any form. Additional safeguards are extended to children and incarcerated/institutionalized persons.

Disaster victims clearly comprise an extremely vulnerable population, depending upon the intensity of their exposure, the trauma they have sustained, and their circumstances at the point they are asked to participate in a research effort. Adherence to the principles of privacy and informed consent comprise an essential minimum. It is our conviction that field research, in the immediate post-disaster period, additionally needs to carefully complement the relief effort. Field researchers should know the available sources for aid and should be prepared to refer participants to appropriate resources. Field researchers should be prepared to be directly helpful in certain circumstances; for example, offering a ride, or making a telephone call. Field researchers should take social action (e.g., reporting, publicizing, pressing the emergency assistance bureaucracy) to assist in rectifying circumstances they may encounter, such as public health hazards. In quantitative studies, field researchers should understand the difference between standardized data collecting and supportive listening and strive to iterate both, with the integrity of the data and the well-being of the subject equally regarded.

The policies of the Federal Emergency Management Agency (FEMA) reflect these ethical considerations following a disaster. FEMA resources are not to be diverted from direct services to disaster victims and FEMA clients' privacy is to be guaranteed, not simply protected by confidentiality/anonymity assurances. Specifically, FEMA-funded programs may not provide researchers with access to their clients, and staff of FEMA-funded programs may not engage in research tasks and activities during working hours in the FEMA program. Hence, disaster research participants need to be identified through other avenues, and academics involved as staff in FEMA-funded enterprises must be careful to conduct research only when not functioning in a FEMA-related role (Garrity, 1993).

Disaster Information Sources

Social and behavioral disaster research is a relatively small enterprise compared with other areas of research activity. Five steps will introduce researchers to what is arguably the mainstream of social work-relevant disaster study. At the federal level, within SAMHSA, the Center for Mental Health Services provides information on disaster mental health services. Within NIH/NIMH, the Violence and Traumatic Stress Research Branch, Traumatic Stress Research Program can also supply needed information. At the University of Colorado at Boulder, the Natural Hazards Research and Applications Information Center is a clearinghouse for disaster information generated by multiple disciplines and offers a bi-monthly publication, *The Natural Hazards Observer*, along with Internet access. At Texas A&M University, the Hazard Reduction and Recovery Center publishes a wide variety of disaster studies emphasizing mitigation and recovery. At the University of Delaware, the Disaster Research Center makes available a publications list with emphasis on social and behavioral studies.

On the Internet, Gopher and WWW searches will reveal a host of on-line resources and reports relating to disasters, including NSF grant information, the Natural Hazards Research Center, and various files on specific disasters and disaster response. PILOTS, the Published International Literature on Traumatic Stress, is a compilation of the literature on the psychosocial, psychological, and behavioral aspects of disasters. PILOTS is part of the Dartmouth College Library On-Line System (DCLOS), is free of charge, and requires no password.

CONCLUSION

This article offers a "blueprint for research readiness" to social work researchers that is intended to position them for important roles in research of the effects of natural or technological disasters. Based on contemporary models of stress research, an overarching conceptual framework is suggested for its capability to guide disaster-focused social work research at the micro, mezzo, and macro levels. Founded in large measure on experience gained in the aftermath of Hurricane Andrew in Miami, Florida in 1992, potential research themes, needs, strategies, and opportunities are identified.

Social work researchers are exhorted to be poised in the event of a disaster and to consider the many unanswered questions surrounding disaster as a focus of *both* planning and inquiry for interim and mitigation phases. The position that academic institutions occupy in society allows them a separate, potentially more objective, vantage point from that of front line service delivery organizations. This "outsider" position can offer important stability to conduct much-needed research in the chaotic situations following natural disasters. Additionally, many agency settings are research capable and strategically positioned to conduct investigations centering on their clients. However, for both academic and agency settings, it is critical that disaster research planning be a priority in times that are free of a specific disaster's anticipated arrival or immediate aftermath, and that these plans and their associated methods be reviewed frequently to maintain their currency.

REFERENCES

Ager, R.D. & Zakour, M.J. (1995, March) Network exchange and the coordination of disaster relief services. Paper presented at the Annual Program Meeting of the Council on Social Work Education, San Diego, CA.

American Red Cross (1993). Disaster services regulations and procedures, ARC 3077-1A.

Applebaum, R.P. (1990). Counting the homeless. In J. Momeni (Ed.), *Homelessness in the United States: Data and Issues*, New York: Praeger. pp. 1-16.

Baum, A. (1987). Toxins, technology, and natural disasters. In G.R. VandenBos and B.K. Bryant (Eds.), *Cataclysms, Crises, and Catastrophes: Psychology in Action*. Washington, D.C., American Psychological Association. pp. 9-53.

Centers for Disease Control (1992). Preliminary report: Medical examiner reports of deaths associated with Hurricane Andrew. *Morbidity and Mortality Weekly Report, 41*(34), 641-644.

Cherry, A. L. & Cherry, M.E. (1995, March) Research as social action in the aftermath of Hurricane Andrew. Paper presented at the Annual Program Meeting of the Council on Social Work Education, San Diego, CA.

Derogatis, L. (1982). Self-report measures of stress. In L. Goldberger & S. Breznitz (Eds.), *Handbook of stress: Theoretical and clinical aspects* (pp. 270-294). New York: The Free Press.

Dynes, R.R. & Tierney, K.J. (Eds.). (1994). *Disasters, collective behavior and social organization*. Newark, DE: University of Delaware Press.

Elliott, G., & Eisdorfer, C. (Ed.). (1982). *Stress and human health: Analysis and implications of research*. New York: Springer Publishing Co.

Freedy, J.R., Resnick, H.S. & Kilpatrick, D.G. (1992). Conceptual framework for evaluating disaster impact: Implications for clinical intervention. In J.H. Gold (Series Ed.) & L.S. Austin (Vol. Ed.), Clinical practice: Vol. 24. *Responding to Disaster* (pp. 3-23). Washington, DC: American Psychiatric Press.

Gillespie, D.F., Sherraden, M.W., Streeter, C.L. & Zakour, M.J. (1986). Mapping networks of organized volunteers for natural hazard preparedness, #PB87-182051/A09. Springfield, VA: National Technical Information Service.

Goldberger, L., & Breznitz, S. (1982). Stress research at a crossroads. In L. Goldberger & S. Breznitz (Eds.), *Handbook of stress: Theoretical and clinical aspects* (pp. 1-6). New York: The Free Press.

Green, B.L. (1993). Mental health and disaster: Research review. Report to NIMH, Requisition 91mf175040. Washington, DC: Georgetown University Medical Center, Department of Psychiatry.

Green, B.L. (in press). Traumatic stress and disaster: Mental health effects and factors influencing adaptation. In E. LieMac & C. Nadselson (Eds.) & J.R.T. Davidson & A. McFarlane (Section Eds.), *International Review of Psychiatry*. Washington, DC: APA Press & the American Psychiatric Association.

Lazarus, R., & Folkman, S. (1984). Stress, appraisal, and coping. New York: Springer Publishing.

Myers, D. (1991). As cited in Green, B.L. (1993). The application of research findings to the planning and operation of mental health services programs following major disasters: Informational needs of service planners, practitioners, and administrators. Unpublished.

Quarantelli, E.L. (1992). Disaster research. In E. Borgatta & M. Borgatta (Eds.), *Encyclopedia of sociology* (pp. 492-498). New York: Macmillan.

Quarantelli, E.L. (1990). Thirty years of catastrophe research. In P. Lagadec (Ed.), *States of emergency: Technological failures and social destabilization* (pp. 222-231). London: Butterworth Heinemann.

Quarantelli, E.L. (1987). Disaster studies: An analysis of the social historical factors affecting the development of research in the area. *International Journal of Mass Emergencies and Disasters*, *5*, 285-310.

Rogge, M.E. (1995, March). Reducing community vulnerability to technological and natural hazards: Tools for empowerment. Paper presented at the Annual Program Meeting of the Council on Social Work Education, San Diego, CA.

Sarafino, E. (1990). *Health psychology: Biopsychosocial interactions*. New York: John Wiley & Sons.

Sieber, J.E. (1992). *Planning Ethically Responsible Research: A Guide for Students and Internal Review Boards*. Newbury Park, CA: Sage.

Predictors of Rural Community Survival After Natural Disaster: Implications for Social Work Practice

Paul Sundet
Joanne Mermelstein

SUMMARY. The Great Flood of 1993 not only devastated much of the midwest, it profoundly changed the social fabric of hundreds of river communities. Why some survived and others did not and the relationship of those outcomes to classic crisis intervention theory is the subject of this year-long qualitative study of eight representative Missouri towns. *[Article copies available for a fee from The Haworth Document Delivery Service: 1-800-342-9678. E-mail address: getinfo@haworth.com]*

INTRODUCTION

The Nature of the Problem

The midwestern Great Flood of 1993 was a natural disaster of horrifying proportions. It submerged 17,000 square miles of land, drove tens of thousands of people from their homes and ultimately

Paul Sundet and Joanne Mermelstein are Associate Professors, School of Social Work, University of Missouri-Columbia, 701 Clark Hall, Columbia, MO 65211.

[Haworth co-indexing entry note]: "Predictors of Rural Community Survival After Natural Disaster: Implications for Social Work Practice." Sundet, Paul and Joanne Mermelstein. Co-published simultaneously in *Journal of Social Service Research* (The Haworth Press, Inc.) Vol. 22, No. 1/2, 1996, pp. 57-70; and: *Research on Social Work and Disasters* (ed: Calvin L. Streeter and Susan A. Murty) The Haworth Press, Inc., 1996, pp. 57-70. Single or multiple copies of this article are available for a fee from The Haworth Document Delivery Service [1-800-342-9678, 9:00 a.m. - 5:00 p.m. (EST). E-mail address: getinfo@haworth.com].

caused $12 billion worth of damage (Erikson, 1993). The flood was truly a "500 year" calamity (U.S. Senate Hearings, July 16, 1993). It also offered an important, albeit unwelcome, opportunity to continue the investigation into rural community survival factors that has been a major research thrust of students and faculty at the University of Missouri-Columbia for the past fifteen years (Bullock, 1986; Hassinger, 1994; Heffernan and Heffernan, 1986; O'Brien, Hassinger, Brown & Pinkerton, 1991). For many of the river towns and rural communities of the corn belt, the flood was not just an isolated, unexpected and overwhelming stressor punctuating the rhythmic flow of normal community processes. In rural communities throughout the Missouri and Mississippi river basins the flood was yet another in a decade-long, cumulative, economic and social challenge to durability. The restructuring of the rural economy, spawned initially by the farm crisis, had taxed the core of community vitality. Institutions, citizen leadership and the corporate will to survive had been severely tested and eroded by successive waves of economic pressure (Albrecht, Murdock, Schiflett, Hamm, Leistritz & Ekstrom, 1988). Many communities have already faded or evaporated under these pressures, but some not only survive but flourish. The reasons for such differential responses are the subject of on-going debate among academics and practitioners alike. Several disciplines have contributed their unique perspective to "survival studies." Community development has focused on group process and cohesiveness, economics on production-distribution-consumption linkages and rural sociology on social system cohesiveness. The special contribution of social work to these efforts has been in the application of crisis theory to the rural community (Sundet & Mermelstein, 1988; Zeller 1986; Sundet & Mermelstein, 1984).

The Flood Crisis and Community Survival: Theory Implications

The physical transformation of place combined with the devastating losses from the '93 flood was profoundly disorienting for victims, emergency crews and volunteers. According to crisis theory, the resulting massive psychic trauma clearly fits the definition of a hazardous event that provoked a crisis state for numerous individuals (Aguilera, 1970; Golan, 1978; Parad, 1965). This impact of the trauma on individuals was the focus of disaster intervention by numerous voluntary and governmental agencies and remained the central concern of a massive mental health and social services effort for 18 months post-flood. A well-researched and documented literature assisted social work professionals in adapting generic crisis knowledge and skills to disaster intervention with micro-systems (Blaufarb & Levine, 1972; Bolin, 1976; Farberow, 1990; Farberow & Gordon, 1986; Freedy, Shaw, Jarrell & Masters, 1992; Kliman, 1976; Newman, 1976).

However, there were community as well as individual survival implications of this crisis as well. Central to crisis theory is the notion that the hazardous event is subjectively perceived by the client as either a threat, loss or a challenge and that depending upon that perception, the actions taken to respond are significantly different. Our prior research in the rural environment led to the hypothesis that the flood-produced trauma, defined as a situational crisis, would have differential meanings among the stricken communities and that a range of community perceptions and responses to the disaster from the proverbial "last straw" to accepting a challenge that finally could be won, could be anticipated.

The assessment protocol used to measure community response focused on nine major dimensions drawn from an interdisciplinary viewpoint of community. The four perspectives of demography, ecology, history and culture are augmented by study of the five community sub-systems that comprise a complete community: government, business and industry, education, religion and health and welfare (Fellin, 1987; Poplin, 1979).

Demography includes a large variety of population descriptors, all of which are found in census analyses. Hypothesized to be of particular relevance in disaster were community size, educational attainment of the populace, age/distribution, community longevity, housing ownership, family income and the poverty rate (Herbers, 1986; Murdock, Potter, Ham, Backman, Albrecht & Leistritz, 1988).

History of rural communities is a complex dimension that informs interpretation of a community's present behaviors. The history of intergovernmental relations, internal strife, coping methods in previous disasters, common heritage, the age of the community and the prior record of horizontal integration of community systems are demonstrably relevant to the nature of community disaster response (Davidson, 1991; Herrick, 1986).

Culture embraces community traditions, individual/group value orientation, common mores, homogeneity of values, ethnocentrism, permeability of the community boundaries vis á vis its dominant culture and survival skill level of the populace (see Etzioni, 1993 and Arendt, 1993 for recent treatments of rural culture).

Ecology includes four major aspects of community: transportation systems, communication mechanisms, land utilization (how land resources are used and developed by the community) and general topography of the land. In this instance, proximity of the community to external resources was considered relevant as well (Fitchen, 1991; Robinson 1990).

METHODOLOGY

Nature of the Study

The study consisted of qualitative case investigation of eight severely impacted river towns in Missouri conducted by graduate social work students and the authors. It was designed to take advantage of the convergence of data sources, opportunity for immediate and repeated access to sites and available student personnel.

Personnel Preparation and Site Selection

According to the U.S. Corps of Engineers, seventy-five communities of all sizes in nine mid-western states suffered "substantial damage" in the flood of '93. The eight chosen for study here are representative of the non-urban towns (500-1200 population) in that group. Besides proximity, selection criteria used included comparable size and institutional structure, Federal Emergency Management Administration (FEMA) designation as Category 1 Impact Communities (i.e., major/severe damage and eligible for maximum aid) and baseline data available from previous studies. Assisting in community selection and used as consultants throughout the study were the members of the University of Missouri Flood Disaster Task Force, a panel of experts from all the relevant colleges and schools of the university established to consult with state government and communities on flood issues.

Graduate social work students in a course in community processes were assigned to 3-5 person teams under immediate supervision of an instructor. The student teams received five weeks of intensive classroom instruction on community and rural sociology, a standardized protocol of community assessment and operational definitions of the nine variables noted above. They were also instructed in conventional case study methods, tools and repositories of relevant data (Patton, 1990). Interview schedules were developed and a field note system devised. In addition and consonant with social work professional values and in anticipation of their encounters with flood victims in the study process, the students were briefed on disaster resources, eligibility criteria and how to access them.

Preliminary Reports of the Field Studies

On-site data gathering began approximately seven weeks after the flood's initial strike in the state. At semester's end after approximately 12 weeks in the field (five months post-initial flood impact on the communities), each student team reported its findings in summary form and in a marathon 5-hour feedback session before their peers, the instructors and members of the Flood Disaster Task Force who provided augmentive feedback that enhanced reliability and validity of the data and facilitated a more complete and coherent synthesis of each assessment. This session was audio-taped for subsequent analysis.

Data Analysis

Subsequent to this initial feedback session, the authors compiled and standardized community profiles and developed a preliminary typology of community flood responses. A variety of data analysis techniques were applied including content analysis and case contrast charts. However, the use of a third technique, a case-ordered effects matrix in which a composite weighted score was assigned to each community based on the semantic set of codes derived from the original field protocol, yielded the most useful results. To permit a longer time frame to judge the communities' recovery outcomes, the authors revisited every town in June, 1994, twelve months post-flood. A description of the community and case analysis matrix at the one-year marker was appended to the original community profile.

Each author independently reviewed the profiles and assigned the cases on a survival continuum. Their respective impressions were then compared, reconciled and externally reviewed by consultants from the Disaster Task Force. Using crisis theory adapted to macro-systems, the authors created a final typology of community outcomes and categorized each community accordingly. Each category was then examined against pre-flood descriptors of the communities. Variables common across categories were identified as predictors of disaster outcomes. Findings and conclusions are discussed below.

FINDINGS AND CONCLUSIONS

Community Dimensions Evaluated

Outcomes for each community were classified as danger or opportunity crisis resolutions. On the opportunity side, communities emerged from the disaster appearing to "Survive and Thrive." On the danger side, some seemed to "Fail and Pale." Three sub-types of failure to thrive were observed within the test communities. These were typified as (1) the annihilated community, (2) the hollow community and (3) the terminal community. Annihilation referred to the permanent and total destruction of all facets of community, physical and intangible. Hollowness referenced a condition of existence as a physical and political entity but barren of effective social organization and psychological dynamism. Determined indifference to the self-destructive processes endemic to community life characterized these towns, foreshadowing their ultimate demise. Terminal described a demoralized community of fractured and missing subsystems, withering vitality in remaining community institutions and diminished capacity and motivation to attend to the regular demands of sustenance.

Predictive/Non-Predictive Variables of Community Survival

Specific, pre-disaster community characteristics were associated with post-disaster survival or failure. The following chart lists the full range of variables examined for their potential relevance to disaster outcome and identifies those variables that actually demonstrated an association with known outcomes. The unique interaction of the significant variables in communities was a major factor in outcome.

Among demographic variables, only the poverty rate appeared to have a strong association with outcome. A pre-existing high poverty rate indicated that residents lacked sufficient resources, even with FEMA loans, to move elsewhere. They were place-bound to a piece of already owned land or a low-tax, low-service locale by virtue of their poverty. Where the poverty rate was fairly high but the town did not survive, other variables existed to mediate its effect.

Dimensions of history that proved predictive were governmental relations, presence of preexisting internal strife in the community and horizontal integration of community subsystems. Where intergovernmental relations were harmonious pre-flood and community subsystems practiced cooperation toward a common interest (usually economic), internal strife tended to be minimal or at least contained and hidden from outsiders. Ecological factors predictive of disaster outcome were communication capacity, topography of the land and proximity to external resources. Communication skills, honed through pre-disaster, intra-community cooperative ventures and economic imperatives such as tourist advertising, were invaluable aids in survival. Communication and survival skills that had enabled "rebel" communities to thwart local pressure on them historically were used to garner helping attention from the larger society despite the negative attitudes of the local governments.

Contrary to expectations, a vibrant economy was not a predictor of community survival. In fact, of the five community subsystems studied in each town, the only one that affected community outcome in disaster was the government. Paradoxically, as governmental authority for many community functions has been centralized at ever higher levels–county, state, federal–local community government in rural areas has been dramatically weakened. In disaster, this

PREDICTIVE AND NON-PREDICTIVE VARIABLES
OF COMMUNITY SURVIVAL

Variable	Predicts	Does Not Predict
Demography		
community size		X
educational attainment		X
age/distribution		X
community longevity		X
housing ownership		X
family income		X
poverty rate	X	
History		
governmental relations	X	
common heritage		X
internal strife	X	
disaster coping		X
age of community		X
horizontal integration	X	
Culture		
community traditions		X
homogeneity	X	
ethnocentricism	X	
permiability	X	
individual/group orientation	X	
common mores	X	
survival skill level		X
Ecology		
transportation		X
communication	X	
land utilization		X
topography	X	
proximity to resources	X	
Government	X	
Business/Industry		X

weakness carried a high cost. Disaster intervention is predicated on intergovernmental emergency management. Relief flows from federal and state to local governments. Applications for community disaster relief had to be made by local officials–most of whom, in rural areas, never anticipated such responsibility. Where city councils or Boards of Trustees were dominated by the affluent majority the minority population was virtually ignored in disaster recovery and left to the ministrations of outsiders. But true heroes emerged as well, as town officials struggled valiantly to subordinate their own sense of loss and emotional upset to the needs of the community. To the extent that their example of leadership and tireless efforts to learn and to respond in the midst of crisis were successful, they are recognized as a major factor in community survival.

IMPLICATIONS FOR RURAL SOCIAL WORK PRACTICE

The practitioner has a dual opportunity and obligation to rural community survival in a disaster situation. The first is to apply the well-tested basic principles of crisis intervention to the immediate situation. The five step process of intervention proposed by Golan (1978) for clinical intervention has applicability at the macro level as well.

Macro Crisis Intervention

1. *Promotes realistic understanding of the event*–in community officials, local caregivers and others who must take charge of disaster recovery. The social worker focuses simultaneously on promoting a realistic assessment of the crisis situation by those who must lead the recovery and, at the same time, constructing channels through which "relevant reality" will be transmitted.

2. *Provides emotional support and hope* that the problems are manageable, that the community leaders and officials are up to the job and will be competent in carrying out their duties. Time must be devoted to officials and caregivers in offering specific guidance, empathy and positive feedback on actions already taken and identification of strengths promotes hope.

3. *Allows/encourages purposeful ventilation*–to relieve key community leaders of their frustration, anger and disappointment in themselves, colleagues or unfulfilled promises of help so that they are free to get on with the job of recovery. Ventilation in brief but frequent doses promotes relief from anxiety, offers self-correction of perceptions and affords the comfort of affective sharing in an emotionally-taxing trauma.

4. *Guides problem partialization*–as civic officials and citizen leaders are inundated with a massive array of problems-to-be-solved. Problem partialization requires prioritization of effort informed by a sound appreciation of the continuously emerging needs and barriers characteristic of disaster.

5. *Assists governmental and human service providers to make a specific plan of action* on an hourly, daily or several-day schedule as the recovery progresses and tensions begin to subside. Attentive to the emotional and behavioral cues in key officials, the social worker knows how to gauge interventions according to the ever-fluctuating capacity of others to accept and make use of them.

Crisis and Disaster Preparedness

The second arena of duty and opportunity also parallels individual crisis intervention. Just as in clinical practice it is the duty of the therapist to assist the client to grow from the experience, it is the responsibility of the macro practitioner to assist the community in developing its capacity to respond to crisis situations in the future. Disaster preparedness, based on the findings and conclusions of this study, is not an isolated, locality-relevant function distinct from community structures and systems. It is part and parcel of community processes and must be addressed as such in a preventive approach.

Based on these principles, the rural social worker who would support community viability, in disaster or otherwise, should:

1. *Build community coalitions*–to promote horizontal integration of community subsystems and to encourage embrace of the cultural and demographic diversity intrinsic to the community. Coalitions designed to coordinate human service delivery greatly enhance the

efficiency and effectiveness of normal rural helping processes but they are the bedrock of swift disaster responsiveness.

2. *Educate the community about mutual support*–when the source of stress is immutable and the conditions of stress are continuous for an indefinite length of time, the capacity to endure and to triumph is bolstered and enriched by the experience of caring and sharing through mutual support. This mediating experience of belonging forms the essence of the psychological or spiritual meaning of community.

3. *Develop communication linkages among critical leaders*–leaders who know each other on a first name basis, understand generally what each does in her/his job, and have an assessment of the other's style, competence, liabilities and resources will cooperate more effectively in the daily business of community life as well as in disaster. Vertical communication among local leaders and officials in extra-local organizations that serve the community is as important as horizontal communication within the community.

4. *Foster resource awareness and preparation*–In the Great Flood, even the most knowledgeable rural human service providers, let alone rural governmental officials, were unfamiliar with the primary disaster relief organizations and how they operate (see Myers, 1944 for a partial list). Generating electronic and print resource directories, training in the who, what, how, and when of disaster-specific access, and creating structures and support for local control and coordination of service delivery are all viable methods of meeting this community need.

5. *Encourage anticipation of and planning for community crises*–knowledge of crisis behavior and crisis intervention is helpful to any community leader or resident, but beyond this core knowledge, leaders in community subsystems should plan how to interface with other community systems if disaster impends. Delegation of responsibilities, allocation of personnel and resources and other key disaster recovery tasks can be anticipated and planned for in advance.

CONCLUSION

The human services literature brilliantly analyzes individual human behavior responses to crisis associated with natural disasters

(Drabek and Biggs, 1968; Fritz and Williams, 1957; Heffron, 1977; and Wenger, 1978). The practitioner can find help with strategies (Lysad, 1985; Myers, 1994; and Tuckman, 1973), techniques (Borgman, 1977; Harshbarger, 1974; and Mitchell, 1983) and material tools (Cohen, Culp & Genser, 1987; Farberow, 1990; Farberow & Gordon, 1986; Hartsough, Resnik & Parad, 1976; and Tierney & Baisden, 1979) to facilitate a positive crisis resolution in disaster victims.

This study, however, directs attention to the macro-system response to disaster. By identifying factors that significantly impacted the disaster responses of communities and their ability to survive, it offers empirical justification for interventive efforts in rural communities that extend far beyond clinical treatment and individual social support considerations. Further, it suggests potential preventive activities leading to community survival are both feasible and effective.

REFERENCES

Aguilera, D.C., Messick, J. and Farrell, M. (1970). *Crisis intervention: Theory and methodology*. St. Louis: C.V. Mosby.

Albrecht, D., Murdock, S., Schiflett, K., Hamm, R., Leistritz, F.L. and Ekstrom, B. (1988). The consequences of the farm crisis for rural communities. *Journal of the Community Development Society*, *19* (2), 119-134.

Blaufarb, H. and Levine, J. (1976). Crisis intervention in an earthquake. *Social work*, *17* (4), 16-19.

Bolin, Robert C. (1976). Family recovery from natural disaster: A preliminary model. *Mass emergencies*, *1* (4), 267-277.

Borgman, R.D. (1977). Crisis intervention in rural community disasters. *Social casework*, *58* (9), 562-567.

Bullock, Bruce. (1986). The farm credit situation: Implications for Agricultural Policy. *Human Services in the Rural Environment*, 10(2), 3-8.

Cohen, R., Culp, C. and Genser, S. (1987). *Human problems in major disasters: A training curriculum for emergency medical personnel*. National Institute of Mental Health, Emergency Services Branch. Washington, DC: U.S. Government Printing Office, DHHS Publication No. (ADM) 90-1505.

Davidson, Osha G. (1991). *Broken heartland: The rise of America's rural ghetto*. New York: Doubleday.

Drabek, T. E. and Biggs, K. (1968). Families in disaster: Reactions and relations. *Journal of marriage and the family*, *30* (8), 403-451.

Erikson, Kai. (1993). After the flood. Columbia (MO) *Daily Tribune*, Sept. 12, 1D.

Etzioni, Amitai. (1993). *The spirit of community*. New York, NY: Crown Publishing Company.

Farberow, N. (Ed.) (1990). *Training manual for human service workers in major disasters. National Institute of Mental Health*. Washington, D.C.: U.S. Government Printing Office, DHHS Publication No. (ADM) 90-538.

Farberow, N. and Gordon, N. (1986). *Manual for child health workers in major disasters*. National Institute of Mental Health. Washington, D.C.: U.S. Government Printing Office, DHHS Publication (ADM) 86-1070.

Fellin, Philip. (1987). *The community and the social worker*. Itasca, IL: Peacock Publishing.

Fitchen, Janet. (1991). *Endangered spaces, enduring places*. Boulder, CO: Westview Press.

Freedy, J., Shaw, D., Jarrell, M. and Masters, C. (1992). Towards an understanding of the psychological impact of natural disasters: An application of the conservation resources stress model. *Journal of traumatic stress*, *5* (3), 441-454.

Fritz, C.E. and Williams, H.B. (1957). The human being in disasters: A research perspective. *The annals of the American academy of political and social science*, *308*, 42-51.

Golan, Naomi. (1978). *Treatment in crisis situations*. New York: The Free Press.

Harshbarger, D. (1974). Picking up the pieces: Disaster intervention and human ecology. *Omega*, *5* (1), 55-59.

Hartsough, D.M., Resnik, H.L.P., and Parad, H.J. (1976). Community resources for disaster aid: An annotated inventory. In Parad, H.J., Resnik, H.L.P. and Parad, L.C. (eds.), *Emergency and disaster management: A mental health sourcebook*. Bowie, MD: Charles Press, 385-91.

Hassinger, Edward. (1994). Settlement patterns and provision of services in the north central region. In David O'Brien (ed.) *A research agenda for studying rural public service alternatives in the north central region*. Ames, IA: North Central Center for Rural Development, Iowa State University.

Heffernan, J. and Heffernan, W. (1986). When farmers have to give up farming. *Rural development perspectives*, *2(3)*, 10-14.

Heffron, E.F. (1977). Interagency relationships and conflict in disaster: The Wilkes-Barre experience. *Mass emergencies*, *2* (2), 111-119.

Herbers, John. (1986). *The new heartland: America's flight beyond the suburbs and how it is changing our future*. New York, NY: Times Books.

Herrick, James. (1986). Farmers revolt! Contemporary farmers' protests in historical perspective: Implications for social work practice. *Human Services in the Rural Environment*, *10(1)*, 6-11.

Kliman, Ann. (1976). The Corning flood project: Psychological first aid following a natural disaster. In Parad, Howard J. (Ed.), *Emergency and disaster management: A mental health sourcebook*. Bowie, MD: The Charles Press, 325-335.

Lysad, Mary (ed.). (1985). *Innovations in mental health services to disaster victims*. Rockville, MD: U.S. Department of Health and Human Services, PHS, ADAMHA, National Institutes of Mental Health. U.S. Government Printing Office, #ADM 85-1390.

Mitchell, J.T. (1983). When disaster strikes. . . . The critical incident stress debriefing process. *Journal of emergency medical services, 8*, 36-39.

Murdock, S., Potter, L., Ham, R., Backman, K., Albrecht, D. and Leistritz, F. (1988). The implications of the current farm crisis for rural America. In S. Murdock and F. Leistritz (eds.), *The farm financial crisis: Socioeconomic dimensions and implications for producers and rural areas*. Boulder, CO: Westview Press.

Myers, Diane (1994). *Disaster response and recovery: A handbook for mental health professionals*. Rockville, MD: U.S. Department of Health and Human Services, PHS, SAMHSA, Center for Mental Health Services. DHHS #(SMA) 94-3010.

Newman, C. Janet. (1976). Children of disaster: Clinical observations at Buffalo Creek. *American journal of psychiatry, 133* (3), 306-312.

O'Brien, D., Hassinger, E., Brown, R. and Pinkerton, J. (1991). The social networks of leaders in more and less viable rural communities. *Rural Sociology*, 56(4).

Parad, Howard. (Ed.) (1965). *Crisis intervention: Selected readings*. New York: Family Service Association of America.

Patton, M.Q. (1990). *Qualitative evaluation and research methods (2d ed.)*. Newbury Park, CA: Sage Publications.

Poplin, Dennis. (1979). *Communities: A survey of theories and methods of research* (3rd ed). New York, NY: Macmillan Publishing Co.

Robinson, Guy. (1990). *Conflict and change in the countryside*. New York, NY: Belhaven Press.

Sundet, P. and Mermelstein, J. (1988). Community development and the rural crisis: Problem-strategy fit. *Journal of community development society, 19(2)*, 93-107.

Sundet, P. and Mermelstein, J. (1984). Rural crisis intervention. *Human Services in the Rural Environment*, Summer/Fall.

Tierney, Kathleen, J. and Baisden, Barbara (eds.). (1979). *Crisis intervention programs for disaster victims–a source book and manual for smaller communities*. Disaster Research Center, Ohio State University. Washington, D.C.: U.S. Government Printing Office, DHEW Pub. (ADM) 79-675.

Tuckman, Alan. (1973). Disaster and mental health intervention. *Community mental health journal, 9* (2), 151-157.

U.S. Congress. Senate Committee on Agriculture, Nutrition and Forestry. (1993). Flood and disaster relief in the midwest: Committee hearings on the scope and components of federal disaster relief in the flood ravaged midwest. U.S. Senate, 103rd Congress, first session. Washington D.C.: U.S. Government Printing Office, #93-0688-P, 103-197.

Wenger, D.E. (1978). Community response to disaster: Functional and structural alternatives. In Quarantelli, E.L. (ed.), *Disasters: Theory and research*. Beverly Hills, CA: Sage Publications, 17-48.

Zeller, Simon. (1986). Grieving for the family farm. *Human Services in the Rural Environment*, 10(2), 27-29.

Research as Social Action in the Aftermath of Hurricane Andrew

Andrew L. Cherry
Mary Elizabeth Cherry

SUMMARY. A study conducted 14 months after Hurricane Andrew examined the long term impact of this natural disaster on the homeless in the hardest hit areas of South Florida. The effects of a natural disaster on the homeless has not been studied in the past. In addition, this study is presented to illustrate a model of social action research. The foundations for the principles of this model are rooted in the best scientific and social justice traditions. The principles are introduced and described using research methodologies that were utilized in this disaster study. How the findings contributed to changes in policy, procedure, and practice are highlighted. *[Article copies available for a fee from The Haworth Document Delivery Service: 1-800-342-9678. E-mail address: getinfo@haworth.com]*

On August 24, 1992, South Florida was hit by Florida's worst and most expensive hurricane ever, inflicting $30 billion in damages. After winds of over 150 mph which caused 40 deaths and seriously damaged more than 75,000 homes, most of the victims in the "hit

---

Andrew L. Cherry is Professor, Barry University School of Social Work, 11300 Northeast Second Avenue, Miami Shores, FL. Mary Elizabeth Cherry is Executive Director, The Biscayne Institute, Miami, FL.

This article is based on a paper presented at the Council on Social Work Education's Annual Program Meeting, San Diego, CA, March 1994.

[Haworth co-indexing entry note]: "Research as Social Action in the Aftermath of Hurricane Andrew." Cherry, Andrew L. and Mary Elizabeth Cherry. Co-published simultaneously in *Journal of Social Service Research* (The Haworth Press, Inc.) Vol. 22, No. 1/2, 1996, pp. 71-87; and: *Research on Social Work and Disasters* (ed: Calvin L. Streeter and Susan A. Murty) The Haworth Press, Inc., 1996, pp. 71-87. Single or multiple copies of this article are available for a fee from The Haworth Document Delivery Service [1-800-342-9678, 9:00 a.m. - 5:00 p.m. (EST). E-mail address: getinfo@haworth.com].

zone" found themselves homeless or living in damaged homes. More than a million people were without electricity, telephone, and water. The temperatures were in the mid-90s during the day and mid-80s at night (Clifford, Leen, & Doig, 1992, December 20).

The following study of the homeless person's "struggle for room and food" (Malthus, 1798) after a major natural disaster is presented to provide information about the impact of a disaster on the homeless, and to illustrate a model of social action research in a disaster setting. The model proposed in this paper is designed to help fulfill our professional commitment to science and social justice by utilizing the best scientific research methodologies available to describe observable phenomena, in this case, related to the recovery of homeless disaster victims.

Fourteen months after Hurricane Andrew (November, 1993), a study was conducted in the hardest hit areas of South Florida to examine the plight of the homeless during the recovery period. In this account of recovery, more than a year after the disaster, local homeless advocates were maintaining that many of the very poor, near homeless, and homeless had been under-served and were at-risk of being forgotten once the majority of the more financially stable individuals and families were situated in housing. A literature review supported their assertions. Vulnerable populations had faced prolonged recovery periods after other disasters.

Much of the disaster research before the 1990s seems to have focused on organization and community preparedness and response (Drabek & Haas, 1969; Dynes, 1967; Stallings, 1973; Yutzy, 1970), the social problems of adjustment and relocation (Dynes & Quarantelli, 1966; Quarantelli, 1984), and disaster/crisis management (Anderson, 1969; Ponting, 1972; Quarantelli, 1983). Since the late 1980s, disaster research has for the most part focused on the response of individuals and groups to the trauma of the experience of a disaster. These studies typically are related to Post-Traumatic Stress Disorder (Green, Kovol, Grace & Vary, 1991; Steinglass & Gerrity, 1990; Van Den Bergh & LeVine-Mann, 1995).

Throughout the past 30 years, there also has been a growing number of studies that reported on the differential impact of a disaster on vulnerable populations (Dynes, 1967; Forrest, 1973; Mann, 1993; Quarantelli, 1979), and specifically how disasters impact such groups as the elderly (Krause, 1987; Phifer & Norris, 1989; Rolin & Klenow, 1988), children (Green, Kovol, Grace & Vary, 1991; Seroka, Knapp, Knight & Siemon, 1986; Udwin, 1993), families (Soloman, Bravo, Rubio-Stipec & Canino, 1993; Wenger, 1987), and racial groups (Dynes, 1988; Roth, 1970). It was believed that a study of homeless victims of a major hurricane would add to this body of knowledge. The effects of a major disaster on the homeless had not been studied.

This project was undertaken because there was an urgent need for a count of homeless people living in the hardest hit areas. The Federal Emergency Management Agency (FEMA) recovery officials were planning to discontinue individual disaster services because they estimated that there were only 300 people who remained homeless in the area. Local relief workers and advocates for the homeless estimated that larger numbers of people were homeless and remained homeless as a result of the hurricane (Garvin, 1993). Additionally, Homestead Air Force Base, a military installation destroyed by Hurricane Andrew, was being decommissioned and fell under the McKinney Act. If a sizable body of homeless people lived in the area, under the McKinney Act the Federal land use plan would give first option on the facility to provide services to the homeless (Rogers, 1995, May 13).

From a research perspective, a study 14 months after a major disaster could have both explanatory and predictive value related to disaster recovery among the homeless. From a social justice perspective, such a study could help empower the homeless and their advocates by giving them evidence to make a stronger case for the need for continued and additional services for the homeless disaster victims.

The over-arching research question for this study focused on relief policies and practices that could have a positive or negative impact on homeless people after a major natural disaster. The research objective was to portray the experience of survival and recovery of the homeless victims during the 14 months that followed Hurricane Andrew. In addition, a count was needed to establish the sampling frame and to produce an accurate count of the homeless living in the recovery area. This count was information needed by both homeless advocates and neighborhood groups who were opposed to homeless services being provided at the closed military facility. The neighborhood groups did not believe there were enough homeless in their community to warrant establishing a homeless service center. More specifically the research questions were:

1. Who are the homeless after the hurricane?
2. What resources and services were available to the homeless after the hurricane?
3. What services facilitated the homeless in their efforts to reestablish themselves in some type of traditional housing after the hurricane?
4. How did the hurricane affect programming and services that had been provided for the homeless prior to the hurricane?

SOCIAL ACTION RESEARCH

The historical tradition of social service and social work research has its foundations in the large-scale social reform movements that took place in the United States during the first 30 years of the twentieth-century. Sociologists and social workers conducted research that was intended to help effect social change, and in many cases it did.

Inspired by the success and social reform brought about by social surveys conducted in London, England by Charles Booth (1840-1916), the Pittsburgh Survey directed by Paul U. Kellogg (1879-1958) was used to collect and disseminate statistics on income, crime, disease, etc., in Pittsburgh from 1906 to 1914. The success of this type of community social survey stimulated the "survey movement" and early social work research (Polansky, 1975a).

The settlement house surveys, which were far less encompassing than the larger community surveys, were motivated by direct contact and a one-to-one familiarity with the people who lived in the communities around the settlement houses. The settlement house surveys, like the larger community surveys, were helpful if not instrumental in promoting social reforms in such areas, for example, as child welfare, labor, and sanitation (Tyson, 1995).

However, by the 1930s, the survey movement had lost its impact and credibility; " . . . it was easy to demonstrate for the umpteenth time that all sorts of social problems tended to be concentrated in the same part of town" (Polansky, 1975a, p. 11). Even more wearisome, these community studies " . . . added little to what practitioners already knew" (Polansky, 1975a, p. 11).

While social work and social service research was stagnant during this period and had lost much if not all of its previous status, in other fields such as psychology and the behavioral sciences, the "scientific method" was being embraced and began to produce theory and knowledge grounded in the logical consistency of the new science (Polansky, 1975b). By the late 1940s, Alfred Khan and others in the Social Work Research Group were calling for a model of social work research that would embrace social science theory and empirical research (the scientific method) in the development and validation of social work knowledge (Maas, 1991).

This model did not exclude social action research, but it obliged social work researchers to conduct their inquiry in a scientific way, which meant a value-free or neutral way. One of the primary tasks of the social work researcher under this rubric is to observe facts without letting one's bias influence the findings.

This canon has been difficult for many advocates to accept. As a result, between the 1930s and 1980s there were few models of social action research proposed. Even so, a number of scientific studies were conducted that contributed to social change in such fields as child welfare, mental health, and minority issues.

More recently, however, there have been several specific social action models suggested (Pieper, 1981; Rapp, Shera & Kisthardt, 1993; Wagner, 1991). Although the approaches are clearly advocacy oriented, and the authors pay homage to the concept of empowerment, these models still have several major flaws that will reduce or negate their effectiveness as social action models. One of the major flaws in these models is that they reject the notion that social action research inquiry should be "value-free." Wagner (1991) writes "Unlike much traditional social science research, which seeks to expand knowledge for its own sake, action research is partisan."

According to the model presented in this paper, researchers may be "partisan" but the research they conduct must be "unbiased." Social action research by definition is suspect for bias. To be effective, it should be conducted with as little prejudice as humanly possible. This is the only way to establish and maintain the credibility of the research.

A SOCIAL ACTION RESEARCH MODEL

The model of social action research we are proposing is based on the knowledge that in most situations social science research can serve a dual purpose. On the one hand, it can generate scientific knowledge. On the other hand, it can provide hard, replicative evidence that a problem exists. This is evidence or findings that can be used to advocate for changes in policy and procedures, and in direct practice.

The model of social action research proposed here is a combination of the best aspects of the qualitative and quantitative research approaches. As such, the model adheres to six fundamental principles:

1. The primary purpose for doing the research is to generate knowledge. The focus is on knowledge about and problems among vulnerable populations.
2. The variables that focus on the area of interest are operationalized to be as sensitive to participants, and as unbiased as scientifically and humanly possible.
3. To provide case and class data, a triangulation research approach–using both qualitative and quantitative techniques–is employed as method. This gives a multi-sided view of the phenomena being studied.
4. The methodology and procedures can be easily replicated by other researchers.
5. In general, the scientific quality of the study is able to withstand a critique by other scientists during a legal challenge.
6. The purpose of dissemination is not to assign fault, but to present the research findings as *prima facia* evidence that specific hypothesized conditions (related to vulnerable populations) do or do not exist.

The following case study is an attempt to show how this model of social action research can be employed in a practice setting to advocate for extended disaster relief services for a vulnerable population. In terms of outcome, this study fulfilled the dual purpose of generating knowledge and providing evidence that even after 14 months a sizeable group of vulnerable people were still homeless in the disaster area. Nevertheless, this model should not be judged on the outcome in this case. The model should be judged on its scientific merit and on the clarity of the approach. Outcomes, because of the socio-political climate, will vary. However, an impeccable model and its operations must remain consistent despite the outcome if social action research is to maintain its credibility.

METHODOLOGY

The procedure, data and findings reported here are only a fraction of the information from this broad and comprehensive study. However, because the purpose of this paper is to illustrate a model of social action research for social work after a disaster, the focus will be on the *count* of those who were homeless in the disaster area.

There were four different types of data collected for this study. Data consisted of: (1) key informant interviews, (2) field observations, (3) a count of the number and location of the homeless, and (4) data from 129 interviews with homeless individuals. This is a data-gathering approach that is often called *triangulation*. It is the process of gathering several different but related types of current data on the same variables to answer questions which no one data-gathering approach can do adequately by itself (Marlow, 1993).

Procedure

To begin the study a team of two trained staff persons interviewed the heads of agencies and groups that provided services to the homeless before and after the hurricane. The interviews used open-ended questions and provided essential qualitative information. By asking the homeless providers what services they provided the homeless after the disaster, and by asking the homeless what help they received and who helped them, beginning details of what was provided the homeless in the disaster area over 14 months were compiled.

To do the count, make the field observations, and conduct the interviews, five additional teams of two surveyors each were trained to canvass the hardest hit disaster areas. These areas stretched from south of Downtown Miami to south of Homestead, Florida, and from the Atlantic Ocean to the Everglades National Park. These areas, approximately 400 square miles, covered the eastern tip of South Florida. It was a mix of suburban areas and large farm operations.

Each of the five teams was composed of one master level student enrolled in the Barry University School of Social Work and one ex-homeless person. The members of the teams were racially and ethnically representative of the homeless in the community. One member of each team spoke Spanish.

The target area was mapped off into grids. As the teams identified homeless individuals, the number of homeless people at the location was noted on a map in the approximate area where the homeless person(s) resided. Each grided area was covered by the same team twice.

To locate homeless encampments in both the urban and rural areas, service providers were asked for information on known locations. However, each team covered their assigned grid areas twice over a two-week period. Proprietors of small local convenience stores and the 'mom and pop' stores in these areas were questioned about the location of homeless people who shopped at their store. In addition, team members asked the homeless they located for information on other encampments of homeless people. The homeless individuals at the sites also were asked to estimate the number of people who lived there, but who were not present at the time of the count. Using these techniques, the people living at known homeless sites were counted and estimated.

THE COUNT

Counting the homeless is much like seeking the Holy Grail; it is no trivial task under normal conditions. It is methodologically problematic and politically controversial. Advocates want high numbers and city and county administrators want low numbers (Wright & Devine, 1995).

In the early 1980s, estimates of the number of homeless by homeless advocates acquired the reputation of "Lying for Justice" (White, 1992). In some cases, the early counts produced exaggerated large numbers because of a loose and broad definition (Kondratas, 1991). In other cases, the numbers were overstated to bring attention to the problem. However, civil administrators who were expected to cope with the growing ranks of the homeless (but did not want the task) declared that they could not plan or develop policy without adequate numbers with which to plan. It took legitimate scientists a number of years and numerous studies before methodology and homeless numbers were developed that both advocates and administrators could accept.

The principal investigator of this study had been doing studies and counts of the homeless in South Florida since 1988. To allow for comparison with findings over the years and from other studies, the HUD definition of a homeless person was used in this study. Homelessness or homeless individual includes:

1. an individual who lacks a fixed, regular, and adequate nighttime residence; and
2. an individual who has a primary nighttime residence that is:
   a. a supervised publicly or privately operated shelter designed to provide temporary living accommodations (including welfare hotels, congregate shelters, and transitional housing for the mentally ill);
   b. an institution that provides a temporary residence for individuals intended to be institutionalized; or
   c. a public or private place not designed for, or ordinarily used as, a regular sleeping accommodation for human beings.

Individual Interviews

Based on previous studies of the homeless living in the area and the data collected from key informants, we estimated that the field teams would find approximately 400 homeless individuals and families. Considering the time limitations, it was decided that the teams should interview 25% of those found. This would provide a representative sample of at least those identified in the field. Table 1 is provided to help describe the homeless in the area.

The questionnaire was made up of 20 open-ended and close-ended items, and five interviewer observation questions. The items covered information relating to age, gender, education, living situation, family, alcohol and drug treatment needs, etc.

The counts and interviews were done on five (5) different days, the weekend preceding Thanksgiving and the weekend and Monday after Thanksgiving. To avoid duplication (counting or interviewing the same person twice) the field teams asked each individual if s/he had been interviewed at any other time or by any other interviewer from the survey teams.

RESULTS

Results are presented from the analysis of key informant interviews, field observations, and interview data. For the sake of brevity, the findings have been summarized.

TABLE 1. Demographic Characteristics N = 129

CHARACTERISTICS	PERCENTAGES & MEANS
Gender	
Male	105 / 81.4 %
Female	24 / 18.6 %
Average Age	41 years
Standard Deviation for Age	12 years
High School Education or more	30 %
Average Time Homeless	19 months
Standard Deviation for Time Homeless	34 months
Homeless 14 months or Less	70 %
Employed Part-time or Full-time	40 %
Interested in A&D Treatment	37 %
Other Health Problems	22 %

Observations of Homeless Encampments

Immediately after the hurricane, encampments of squatters sprang up throughout the area. These encampments were located in wooded areas and on empty lots surrounding the cities and residential areas. Residents who had been made homeless by the hurricane, people who had been homeless before the disaster, and contract laborers often with families who came into the area for employment and to help rebuild after the hurricane had no other choice but to set up a camp. There was no housing available.

However, by November 1993, when this survey was conducted, the majority of the original campsites had been cleared out by the passing of time and the police. Approximately nine months after the disaster, local authorities began enforcing the ordinance against unlicensed campsites. Abandoned buildings and their adjacent properties that were being used by the homeless, especially government-owned properties, had been fenced in and guards were used to keep out squatters. The residents in the most conspicuous campsites, homeless victims and contract laborers alike, were driven out and their sheds, tents, and temporary homes were torn down.

In far too many of the destroyed buildings, the damage was so extensive that it was dangerous for squatters to live in the damaged structures. However, low income housing was non-existent. Many people left homeless by the hurricane reported having a regular income, in several cases Supplemental Security Income (SSI), but they were unable to find housing at a price they could afford, given the shortage of housing in general in the disaster area.

Estimate of Number of Homeless Persons

The estimate of the total number of homeless persons was based on those who the surveyors were able to physically count plus an estimate of those homeless missed during the street count. Based on the multiplier utilized in this study,[1] it was estimated that the street count missed 66% of the homeless people living in the area. The total number of people counted and estimated was 1,797. This total is derived by multiplying the actual number of homeless people counted (599) times a multiplier of three (3).

The homeless individuals who were missed by this street count were people not in the area when the teams made their two passes. From previous homeless studies in the area, we knew that even on Saturday and Sunday some homeless people would be working on the farms. We also knew that some people would not be recognized as homeless. We knew that for whatever reason, people in many areas would not know that homeless people were living around them. We also had learned that due to the transient nature of life for the homeless person, we would miss a number of people who lived in secluded and hidden sites where they would arrive very late and leave very early. This is where we assume the other 66% of the homeless were when the street count was conducted in November 1994.

Considering the number of people in the disaster area who had been homeless for 14 months or less (70%), one of the logical explanations for their homelessness would have to be the disaster. This percentage suggests that more than a thousand individuals were still homeless, basically as a result of the disaster. The fact that families on welfare and individuals with SSI were still living in make-shift shelters and church tents was testimony to the lack of low income housing available to the poor and homeless in this area 14 months after the hurricane.

DISCUSSION

To be classified as social action research under this model, the research effort must first be good science. The homeless study presented here is offered as an example of how our proposed model of social action research can be implemented. It is by no means perfect, field research rarely is, but it describes an application of the principles of the model.

1. *The primary purpose for doing the research is to generate knowledge. The focus is on knowledge about and problems among vulnerable populations.* The findings from this study added to our knowledge of how a disaster impacts on one of our most vulnerable populations. The findings were useful in helping homeless providers refocus on the homeless in the di-

saster area. The findings of the study provided information that was used to convince FEMA to continue relief efforts for an additional year. The findings also provided support for a successful application to utilize part of the decommissioned Homestead Air Force Base to develop homeless programs.

2. *The variables that focus on the area of interest are operationalized to be as sensitive to participants and as unbiased as scientifically and humanly possible.* This study (especially the count and estimate), although as methodologically problematic as any homeless count done in the last few years, tried to avoid biasing the count one way or the other. It was not rigged to support one side of an issue or the other.

The hypothesis that governed this study was based on the assumption of 'no difference'. In other words, in this study, we began with the expectation that there would be 'no difference' in the number of homeless living in the disaster area and the number that the FEMA relief administrators had estimated.

In this study, we focused the research on areas where vulnerable populations appeared to be experiencing more severe, long-term problems as a result of a major disaster. However, as scientists, we were first committed to gathering information and building knowledge. If the findings supported our cause, excellent. If the findings did not support our cause, we would report the findings anyway. We would possibly re-evaluate our variables and try to devise the next best explanation for the findings, but the findings would still be reported.

3. *To provide case and class data, a triangulation research approach–using both qualitative and quantitative techniques–is employed as method.* In this study, both qualitative and quantitative techniques were employed in the overall design of the study. We were trying to generate as many converging views of the homeless disaster victims as was feasible (triangulation data).

4. *The methodology and procedures can be easily replicated by other researchers.* The procedures used to collect the data could be replicated by advocates and opponents alike. In fact, approximately one year later, the methodology we used to

count the homeless was used in a different part of the county by another homeless advocacy group.

5. *The scientific quality of the study is able to withstand a critique by other scientists during a legal challenge.* In today's legal climate, researchers (especially social action researchers) must be able to defend their methodology and findings in a court of law. The principal investigator was subpoenaed and successfully defended the methodology and findings at two federal trials related to the homeless counts that had been conducted in 1988 and 1989.

6. *The purpose of dissemination is not to assign fault, but to present the research findings as 'prima facia' evidence.* The final report on this study was distributed to local and county officials, homeless providers, and other universities in the state. The report does not blame groups or individuals, but carefully details the number and location of homeless in the disaster areas. It also highlights, with a great deal of accuracy, the plight of the homeless victims after this disaster.

Why get involved in social action research? As social workers, we have little choice. Our profession commits us to the development of knowledge and to the promotion of social justice. However, until recently there were few practical models of social action research described in the literature to help meet these responsibilities. The model presented here, we believe, has promise. With future contributions that will surely be made by others, this model could be configured to produce one or more better models of social action research. These are models that could be viable into the twenty-first century. Like our colleagues, we look forward to having a choice of models that can be used to conduct social action research in the effort to insure equitable treatment even for the most vulnerable of groups.

NOTE

1. The multiplier used in this estimate was developed in earlier studies using a technique called the 'capture, recapture' method (Cherry, 1990). The original multiplier was developed for this area of South Florida in the winter between 1988 and 1992. During that period, emergency homeless shelters were opened on

'cold nights' (temperatures were expected to fall below 35 degrees). This typically occurred two or three times a year.

When the emergency shelters opened, the homeless individuals and families who availed themselves of the emergency shelter were counted. Once counted, this group was viewed as an identified population. The next step was to follow this known group back into the streets and find them a second time. A week after the shelters closed, giving time for the homeless who were in the emergency shelters to reestablish their residency, a street count was conducted to find as many homeless people as possible *who had stayed in emergency shelters*. Although it was a street count, only the homeless who had been in emergency shelters were important for developing the multiplier.

The identification process used during the street count was straightforward. The surveyors went up to every person they thought to be homeless and after explaining that they were from Barry University and helping to conduct a survey, the surveyors asked each person if the person had stayed in an emergency shelter the week before. Consistently, these street counts found only 33% of the homeless who had been in an emergency shelter on a cold night the week before.

This finding was then used to help adjust for those missed during a street count. If 66% of the homeless who were in emergency shelters could not be found in a street count, then the inference is that a street count of all the homeless will also miss 66% of the homeless. Although problematic in many ways, the multiplier is far beyond the educated guess.

REFERENCES

Anderson, W.A. (1969). Social structure and the role of the military in natural disasters. *Proceedings of the 1968 water resources colloquium*. 36-47.

Cherry, A. (1990). "The Magnitude and Nature of Homelessness in South Florida." *The South Florida Homeless Studies*. A Monograph. Barry University Library, Miami Shores, FL. *Vol. 1*.

Clifford, D., Leen, J. & Doig, S.K. (1992, December 20). What went wrong. *The Miami Herald*. p. 16SR.

Drabek, T. & Haas, E.J. (1969). How police confront disaster. *Transaction*. (6) 33-38.

Dynes, R.R. & Quarantelli, E.L. (1966). Effects of disaster on community life, and function of an organization under stress. *Proceedings of seminar on family agencies' role in disaster*. Canadian Department of National Health & Welfare. Nov. 14-17: 3-6, 7-11.

Dynes, R.R. (1967). Societal and community problems in disaster. *EMO National Digest*. (7) 16-18.

Dynes, R.R. (1988). Cross-cultural international research: Sociology and disaster. *International Journal of Mass Emergencies and Disasters*. (6): 101-129.

Forrest, T. R. (1973). Needs and group emergence: Developing a welfare response. *American Behavioral Scientist*. (16) 413-425.

Garvin, G. (1993). Reaping the whirlwind. *Reason*, 24, 26-31.

Green, B.L., Kovol, M., Grace, M.C., & Vary, M.G. (1991). Children and disaster: Age, gender, and parental effects on PTSD symptoms. *Journal of the American Academy of Child and Adolescent Psychiatry*. Vol 30(6): 945-951.

Kondratas, A. (1991). Estimates and public policy: The politics of numbers. *Housing Policy Debate*. 2, 631-647.

Krause, N. (1987). Exploring the impact of a natural disaster on the health and psychological well-being of older adults. *Journal of Human Stress*. Vol 13(2): 61-69.

Maas, H.S. (1991). Still dancing: Review of Helen Harris Perlman's "Looking back to see ahead" and "The dancing clock and other memories." *Readings: A Journal of Reviews and Commentary in Mental Health*. 6, 18-22.

Malthus, T. R. (1798). *An essay on the principle of population as it effects the future improvement of society with remarks on the speculation of Mr. Godwin, M. Condorcet, and other writers*. Republished, NY: Macmillan, Ltd. 1926.

Mann, P. H. (Ed.). (1993, March). *Lessons learned from Hurricane Andrew*. (Available from Florida International University, Miami, FL 33199).

Marlow, C. (1993). *Research methods for generalist social work*. Pacific Grove, CA: Brooks/Cole Publishing Co.

Phifer, J.F. & Norris, F.H. (1989). Psychological symptoms in older adults following natural disaster: Nature, timing, duration, and course. *Journal of Gerontology*. Vol 44(6): 9207-9217.

Pieper, M. (1981). The obsolete scientific imperative in social work research. *Social Service Review*. 56, 146-148.

Polansky, N.A. (1975a). Introduction: Social and historical context. In N.A. Polansky (Ed.) *Social Work Research: Methods for the Helping Profession* (rev. ed.) (pp. 1-17). Chicago, IL: The University of Chicago Press.

Polansky, N.A. (1975b). The design of research. In N.A. Polansky (Ed.) *Social Work Research: Methods for the Helping Profession* (rev. ed.) (pp. 1-17). Chicago, IL: The University of Chicago Press.

Ponting, R.J. (1972). Emergency welfare services in civil disorder. *EMO National Digest*. (12) 11-16, 22.

Quarantelli, E.L. (1979). Some needed cross-cultural studies of emergency time disaster behavior: A first step. *Disasters*. (3) 307-314.

Quarantelli, E.L. (1983). The delivery of disaster emergency medical services: Recommendations from systematic field studies. *Disaster Medicine*. 41-44.

Quarantelli, E.L. (1984). Social problems of adjustment and relocation: Some questions and comments. *Proceedings of the International Conference on Disaster Mitigation Program Implementation*. Ocho Rios, Jamaica. Alexandria VA: Center for international development planning and building, Virginia Polytechnic Institute and State University: 84-90.

Rapp, C.A., Shera, W. & Kisthardt, W. (1993). Research strategies for consumer empowerment of people with severe mental illness. *Social Work*. *38*(6): 727-735.

Rogers, P. (1995, May 13). Homeless shelter site proves hard sell. *The Miami Herald*. pp. 1B, 4B.

Rolin, R.C. & Klenow, D.J. (1988). Older people in disaster: A comparison of black and white victims. *International Journal of Aging and Human Development*. Vol 26(1): 29-43.

Roth, R. (1970). Cross-cultural perspectives on disaster response. *American Behavioral Scientist*. (13) 440-451.

Seroka, C.M., Knapp, C., Knight, S., & Siemon, C. (1986). A comprehensive program for postdisaster counseling. *Social Casework*. Vol 67(1): 37-44.

Soloman, S.D., Bravo, M., Rubio-Stipec, M., & Canino, G.J. (1993). Effect of family role on response to disaster. *Journal of Traumatic Stress*. Vol 6(2): 255-269.

Stallings, R. (1973). The community context of crisis management. *American Behavioral Scientist*. (16) 312-325.

Steinglass, P., & Gerrity, E. (1990). Natural disasters and post-traumatic stress disorder: Short-term versus long-term recovery in two disaster-affected communities. *Journal of Applied Social Psychology*. Vol 20(21, pt.1): 1746-1765.

Tyson, K. (1995). *New foundations for scientific social and behavioral research: The heuristic paradigm*. Needham Heights, MA: Allyn and Bacon.

Udwin, O. (1993). Annotation: Children's reactions to traumatic events. *Journal of Child Psychology & Psychiatry & Allied Disciplines*. 34(2). 115-127.

Van Den Berg, N. & LeVine-Mann, N. (March 1995). *Critical Incident Stress Debriefing: A Practice Method to Reduce Workplace Traumatic Stress*. A conference presentation to be presented at the Council on Social Work Education, 41st Annual Program Meeting.

Wagner, D. (1991). Reviving the action research model: Combining case and cause with dislocated workers. *Social Work*. *36*(6); 477-482.

Wenger, D.E. (1987). Collective behavior and disaster research. *Sociology of Disasters*. (Eds.) R.R. Dynes, B. DeMarchi and C. Pelanda. (Milan, Italy: Franco Angeli): 213-238.

White, R. (1992). *Rude awakenings: What the homeless crisis tells us*. San Francisco, CA: Center for Self Governance.

Wright, J.D. & Devine, J.A. (1995). Housing dynamics of the homeless: Implications for a count. *American Journal of Orthopsychiatry*. 65(3); 320-329.

Yutzy, D. (1970). Priorities in community response. *American Behavioral Scientist*. (13) 344-353.

Community Responses to Chronic Technological Disaster: The Case of the Pigeon River

Hussein H. Soliman

SUMMARY. A case study method was used to examine factors that contribute to community response to chronic technological disaster and to consider the dynamics that evolve within these communities. The Social Process Model (Edelstein, 1988) provided a theoretical framework for the study. Findings provided evidence of multiplicity of impacts regarding the pollution of water resources. Factors influencing community response include history, environmental awareness, economics, and community participation. Considering the longevity of disaster, communities may be forced to try different strategies to minimize its impacts. Community activism represents the most significant strategy in responding to the disaster. *[Article copies available for a fee from The Haworth Document Delivery Service: 1-800-342-9678. E-mail address: getinfo@haworth.com]*

Exposure to toxic waste is a growing problem in the United States and worldwide. Massive increases in the use of chemicals in industry have provided new products for the market; however, such use has also created critical problems. Rural communities report

---

Hussein H. Soliman, PhD, is Assistant Professor, School of Social Work, Southern Illinois University at Carbondale.

Paper presented at the 13th World Congress of Sociology, Bielefeld, Germany, July 18-23, 1994.

[Haworth co-indexing entry note]: "Community Responses to Chronic Technological Disaster: The Case of the Pigeon River." Soliman, Hussein H. Co-published simultaneously in *Journal of Social Service Research* (The Haworth Press, Inc.) Vol. 22, No. 1/2, 1996, pp. 89-107; and: *Research on Social Work and Disasters* (ed: Calvin L. Streeter and Susan A. Murty) The Haworth Press, Inc., 1996, pp. 89-107. Single or multiple copies of this article are available for a fee from The Haworth Document Delivery Service [1-800-342-9678, 9:00 a.m. - 5:00 p.m. (EST). E-mail address: getinfo@haworth.com].

escalating numbers in the incidents of dumping hazardous materials in their land and water resources (Rogge, 1993). This new trend is associated with mounting rates of death, disability, birth defects and cancer (Epstein, Brown, & Pope, 1982). Concurrent research indicates that toxic waste leads to medical, economic, social, and psychological consequences (Bachrach and Zautra, 1983; Edelstein, 1988). Protection from hazardous materials is a new challenge that rural communities face. However, rural communities typically lack the resources that would enable them to fight the trend.

Studies find a consistent relationship between poverty and environmental hazards (Rogge, 1993). Communities suffering the consequences of toxic waste are generally characterized by low socio-economic status, high unemployment rates, high school drop-out rates, and other social problems, such as widespread dependency on governmental social programs and family and community disruption (Edelstein, 1988).

Responses to chronic technological disasters vary from community to community and are determined by many interactive variables. However, research shows that community involvement in the process to fight the disaster seems to be a salient variable. In view of the absence of a comprehensive national environmental policy, community responses are often the only available alternative that people have to deal with these stressful life circumstances.

In an attempt to understand the impact of chronic technological disasters on rural communities, this study explores the multiple factors that influence community responses and methods applied to deal with such a stressor. Accordingly, the study seeks to address the following questions:

1. What are the factors that contribute to community responses to chronic technological disasters?
2. What socio-economic dynamics evolve within a contaminated community involved in fighting chronic technological disasters?

A HISTORY OF PIGEON RIVER POLLUTION

Cocke County, located in eastern Tennessee, is a poor community in the Appalachian mountains. The county seat, Newport, was settled in the late 1800s. This area is characterized by high mountains, beautiful, fertile valleys, numerous cliffs, and three major rivers. Due to the wealth of natural resources in the area, agriculture was the economic base of the community for many years. During the 1930s, the canning industry, established by the Stokely brothers, became one of the major projects in the community, as a variety of crops grew in the region. In addition, mining and lumber industries provided economic support for Cocke County.

The Pigeon River, which is one of the three rivers in this county, flows down from the mountains of the Pisgah Forest, through Haywood County, North Carolina, crosses the Tennessee border in Cocke County, and finally empties into the French Broad River near Knoxville, Tennessee. The first sign of pollution of the Pigeon River occurred in 1908 when a paper mill, Champion International Paper Company, began operations in Canton, North Carolina. Although the mill provided a stable economic base for Haywood County, North Carolina, the waste from the production process has polluted the Pigeon River since production began. The water discharged from the paper mill into the river is colored, hot, has a low level of oxygen, and is contaminated with chemicals. When the mill began production, downstream residents immediately observed a drastic change in the water. It was brown, foamy, and smelled like rotten eggs. This abrupt change in water quality made the water unsafe for drinking and caused a drastic decrease in fish.

Since 1908, conditions of the Pigeon River have been studied by numerous state and federal agencies, including North Carolina and Tennessee, the Tennessee Valley Authority (TVA), and the United States Environmental Protection Agency (EPA). Most studies found a wide variety of pollutants afflicting the waterway. The Pigeon River's waters were chemically, biologically, and aesthetically degraded. A visual observation of the Pigeon River above the mill's discharge point in Canton showed the water to be crystal clear, with rocks visible at a depth of several feet. In contrast, the water below the mill is murky and coffee-colored with foam along the entire length to Douglas Lake, a distance of 64.5 miles.

Throughout the mill's history, Champion officials vigorously responded to accusations regarding polluting the river by maintaining that it was only a color problem. Although reports of the presence of chemicals and highly toxic materials in the water have been published, the company has generally been successful in minimizing these impacts through reports and media coverage filled with technical jargon. For example, when dioxin was found in the fish tissues, Champion declared that a new effort was being made to minimize such discharges. Contrary to Champion's denials, empirical studies continued to show the adverse effects of Champion's discharges on water quality. An assessment of water quality by Schacher (1992) found that the water quality, aquatic plant communities, and the fish population have been severely degraded by the discharge from the Champion mill.

The Socio-Economic and Environmental Conditions of Cocke County

Cocke County has been known as the state's unruly child with a deviant social history, including being known as the nation's moonshine capital. Historically, Cocke County has experienced severe poverty, and residents had few opportunities for stable work. Of the total county population of 29,141, over twenty-five percent live in poverty. As expected in an area of concentrated poverty, there is a lack of adequate health services in the area. Cocke County has a high percentage of low birth weight babies (9.9 percent), correlating with a high infant mortality rate of 13.3 percent. In general, women, infant, and children's health services in Cocke County are inadequate (Erwin, 1991).

In February 1993, there were 2,676 Medicaid cases and 845 Aid to Families With Dependent Children (AFDC) cases. The Department of Human Services indicates that 2,300 persons in Cocke County receive Social Security Income and Medicaid. Also, in February 1990, 25.8 percent of the entire population was receiving food stamps, for a dollar amount of $60,537. This high dependency on government assistance programs presents a critical situation for Cocke County. Any cut in federal assistance would have a devastating impact on families and on the community (Job Service, 1993).

Cocke County is a poor Appalachian community that has historically experienced economic exploitation. Foreign investments were attracted to the area because of its abundant resources. The timber industry was one of the early forms of investments introduced to the community and was characterized by a temporary business base that provided jobs, but no local reinvestment of the profits.

THEORETICAL FRAMEWORK

Research in environmental disasters distinguishes between chronic disaster and acute disaster. This study emphasizes chronic technological disaster. Chronic disaster is characterized by its longevity which produces a particular set of perceptions, impacts and responses. Boss (1987) defines chronic stress as "a situation that runs a long course, is difficult to amend, and has a debilitating effect on the family" (p. 699).

A number of characteristics are used to specify chronic stressor events. These characteristics include: ambiguity versus predictability (where uncertainty regarding the facts about the stressor event is present); the context in which the chronic stressor event develops (whether it is the result of a larger context such as inflation, living near an active volcano, and the closing of a factory, or the result of an individual pathology, such as the continuous illness of a family member); and the visibility of the stressor event, particularly where some events cannot be observed or assessed (Boss, 1987).

Chronic events such as the contamination of a river can be observed through the color of the water and its odor. However, some types of pollution cannot be observed, such as dioxin level. In most cases, the unobservable pollutant can be more harmful than the visible one. The importance of defining the type of stressor was highlighted in Boss's work: "because of the importance of both general characteristics and specific descriptors of chronic stressors, it is essential that researchers identify and describe categorically the events that they are investigating" (p. 699).

The Social Process Model

This study utilizes the Social Process Model in exploring the impacts of technological disasters on the community and the process that determines community responses to such a threat. Edelstein (1988) developed the Social Process Model (Figure 1) to examine technological disasters and their relationship to the social context of communities.

The adoption of the model in this study provides a better understanding of the impact of toxic materials on the individual, the family, and the community. The Social Process Model presents four postulates: (1) the social and psychological impact of toxic exposure involves complex interactions among various levels of society that differ across time and environmental dimensions; (2) these impacts not only affect how victims behave, but how they perceive and comprehend their lives, in both short and long terms; (3) toxic exposure incidents are stressful, forcing victims to adopt some form of coping response; and (4) contamination is inherently stigmatizing and arouses anticipatory fears. The model recognizes that any complex event, such as toxic exposure, has impacts at various levels

FIGURE 1. The Social Process Model

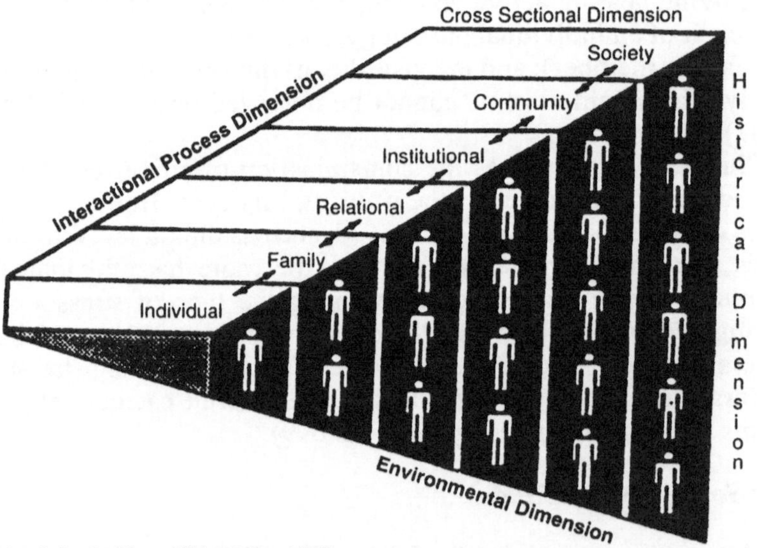

Note: Adapted from Edelstein, 1988

of society both simultaneously and over time. These contexts are examined in light of the historical and environmental dimensions. The historical dimension indicates that groups, organizations, and communities are influenced by specific and relevant past events. The environmental dimension includes both the physical and social environments and how both are affected by toxic exposure. The link between the historical and environmental dimensions is the continuous interaction between the historical realities of the exposure and the present situation of people's lives. Edelstein suggests that the response of an institution to toxic exposure reflects not only the influences of the institution's own history, but also its broader social environment.

Exposure to toxic materials may cause new strains in victims' lives, intensify existing strains, or give new meaning to old problems. The model considers stress as occurring at every level of social process, affecting family, relational, institutional, community, and social dynamics. Accordingly, response to toxic exposure requires a system response rather than an individual response.

METHODOLOGY

This study investigated the aspects of chronic technological disaster using case study analysis based on the review of documents, interviews, non-participant observation and a short survey that measures community members' perceptions and attitudes toward the pollution of the Pigeon River. The use of multiple methods of data collection is suggested by the Social Process Model, which views exposure to toxic materials as multi-dimensional, including impacts on the individual, family, relational, institutional, community, and society dimensions (Edelstein, 1988).

Data Collection

Four steps were utilized in data collection. Initially, 50 structured interviews with activists, officials, scientists, and community members (i.e., school teachers, businessmen, directors of service departments, and media representatives) were conducted, utilizing an interview guide and a coding scale for stress assessment. These interviews were designed to assess community perceptions and attitudes toward the pollution of the Pigeon River in east Tennessee. Other interviews were conducted to collect information about the involvement of different agencies in dealing with the pollution. A number of activists were asked to share their views and discuss their efforts at fighting the pollution. The interview method was helpful in understanding the prolonged process of community involvement with the pollution. Scientists and officials provided technical information about the extent of the pollution and the risk factors involved.

The second method, based on the Social Process Model, involved collecting historical information through the review of archival resources. This historical review of documents was useful in showing different perspectives of the pollution, as well as the influential events which occurred throughout the history of the community. Numerous studies, journal articles, reports, and newspaper articles that explained the history of the pollution of the Pigeon River were inspected. The study of water quality of the river involved data collected from scientific studies conducted by a number of environmental agencies throughout the community history (TVA, 1983; Schacher, 1992).

A short survey was designed to determine community residents' attitudes and perceptions of the problem. The survey was mailed to 84 families that live on the banks of the river with 50 returned or a 59% return rate. The head of the family, to whom the survey was mailed, was instructed to respond to the survey, considering the views of other family members. Finally, observational methods to understand the community dynamics of dealing with the pollution of the river were utilized. Non-participant observation was used to assess community responses during group meetings and activities related to the river. Observation was also used during the class action suit filed by the community residents against Champion International that continued for almost three months in 1992. Content analysis was used to examine different responses of community leaders, activists, families, officials, scientists, and others who participated in non-structured interviews.

RESULTS

Community Responses to Chronic Technological Disaster

A review of hundreds of documents, newspaper articles and interviews suggested the necessity of dividing community responses into three categories. At the beginning of the pollution of the Pigeon River in 1908, residents of Cocke County made individual efforts to complain to different agencies and organizations, including the paper company in Canton, North Carolina. These efforts continued for almost 75 years but were insufficient in achieving change. The formation of a social movement organization known as the Dead Pigeon River Council (DPRC) was the second strategy utilized by the community residents. The DPRC has been successful in gaining attention and increasing public awareness of the problem. Finally, community residents adopted a third strategy–a class action suit.

Early Community Response

Early in this century, the pollution of the Pigeon River took the residents of Cocke County by surprise. The Pigeon River was a critical feature in the community that symbolized the beauty and serenity of the area. When residents of Cocke County observed changes in the water color, they complained to various agencies in Tennessee. Evidence of the pollution was detected and the state of Tennessee became aware of the situation, but lack of funds at that time delayed state efforts to reverse the condition of the river. In January 1912, Governor Hooper of Tennessee granted Champion additional time to perfect the chemical process for the purification of the Pigeon River. A newspaper article at that time reported: "Hooper took the position that the state had no desire to embarrass the Fiber Company but that, if after a practical test the process was found unsatisfactory, then legal means would be taken for the protection of the commonwealth interests" (*The Plain Talk*, January 1912).

This study documents the beginning of political involvement as part of the process of community response. Champion responded to the extension granted by the Governor of Tennessee in 1912 with a promise to build a $750,000 plant that would take care of the pollution. Champion's tactics for facing public and political pressure were characterized by: (1) the public expression of deep concern about the problem; (2) the promise of new technology in the near future but which was seen by concerned citizens as a tactic for gaining time and avoiding further public pressure; (3) the denial of any sort of wrong-doing; (4) the emphasis of the industry's economic value to the region; and (5) attempts to sway public attention through the media in order to forge support. This strategy historically worked for the company due to their ability to allocate funds toward this effort.

Technological promises have made community residents believe in the company's ability to install advanced technology to eliminate the problem. A newspaper article published in September 1923 reported that tons of fish died in the Pigeon River as a result of acid from the mill (*The Plain Talk*, 1923). That was the first time that residents saw the actual impact of the pollution. When people in Cocke County complained of the loss, the company threatened to close the mill and ridiculed the value of fish. In doing so, the company represented the problem as fish versus jobs.

Over the years, that theme has frequently been used by the company whenever residents raised their concerns about the polluted river. For example, when public pressure was heightened in 1980, the company promised that the 1994 completion of a $300 million modernization program would solve the problem. Again, many residents were reassured, as were politicians, government officials, and administrators who granted Champion the time it requested. However, the residents have waited 85 years and the technological promises remain unfulfilled.

Generally, the residents' response to the continuation of the pollution in the river was represented by individual response. Concerned citizens in Cocke County travelled to the mill in Canton, North Carolina to discuss the problem with the company officials. The company typically expressed concern over the issue and promised the visitors that new technology would resolve the problem in the near future.

Organized Community Protest

During the 1970s and 1980s a new environmental movement emerged on the U.S. scene. Incidents of technological disasters such as those at Three Mile Island and Love Canal promoted environmental awareness on the national level. People realized that environmental disasters *can* happen and that their impact is often beyond individual coping capabilities. After Champion failed to fulfill numerous promises, the need for community involvement became important.

The 1986 emergence of the Dead Pigeon River Council (DPRC) marked a new era in the fight against the pollution of the river. After almost eighty years of pollution, the DPRC led the first collective fight against Champion. The official birth of the DPRC was at midnight on December 31, 1986. About 200 Cocke County residents attended a rally on the main bridge in the city of Newport. The pre-mobilization process included advertising in the media, distributing flyers, and personal communication. The organizers rang bells and gave speeches that addressed the community's concerns.

The DPRC succeeded in representing a broad community perspective regarding the pollution of the river. Initially, DPRC's plan was to stage year-round activities to increase community awareness. The DPRC became involved in the discharge permit process, challenging the company to comply with the water standard set by the State of Tennessee. The DPRC was involved in the issuance of the permit and attended meetings with officials in the State of Tennessee, the EPA, and Champion International. The most effective strategy utilized by the DPRC was publicity of the issue through issuing press releases to local, state, and national media.

For the first time, Champion International was faced with a strong and organized opposition from the residents of Cocke County that had challenged the company's position utilizing effective strategies. However, the company continued its battle against Cocke County's efforts to improve the condition of the river. When the EPA took over responsibility for issuing a discharge permit, two public hearings were organized in Asheville, North Carolina and Knoxville, Tennessee. A "gentleman's" agreement between Champion and the DPRC stipulated that no members of the opposing community would attend the hearing held in the other community. Although the Tennessee group upheld their promise, Champion arranged for transportation of its employees to the Knoxville hearings. Fifty buses carried more than 2,000 employees to the hearing. Trust in Champion, which had before been in question, deteriorated further.

On another occasion, the company requested support from the people of North Carolina, threatening that, if the new permit was approved, the company would be forced to close. This threat stirred controversy in North Carolina. Over 180,000 letters were sent to the U.S. EPA Region IV headquarters in Atlanta requesting that no changes be allowed in the discharge permit. The scope of the controversy was expanded with a November 1987 DPRC press conference that presented evidence uncovered by Greenpeace of dioxin in waterways supporting paper mills similar to the one in Canton. Some members of the group and Cocke County officials demanded that the Pigeon River be tested for dioxin. Community concerns were expanded beyond color to include health and public safety issues. The DPRC succeeded in promoting public awareness by utilizing available technology and challenging the technical aspects of the discharge permit. The new movement succeeded in rallying public opinion against a powerful opponent that has managed to control the future of a small community and deny them any access to a clean river.

Community Involvement in a Class Action Suit

The third community response to the pollution began in January, 1991 when 2,600 residents of Cocke County filed a $367.9 million class action suit against Champion. The case was presented to the United States District Court for the Eastern District of Tennessee at Greeneville. According to the Court's record, the charge included the following:

> The plaintiffs claim that Champion International Corporation's pulp and paper mill in Canton, North Carolina, discharged waste water which contains many toxic chemicals into the Pigeon River; that its paper-making process also discolors the river's water and makes it foul-smelling; that Champion's

> use of the river constitutes a nuisance that unreasonably interferes with their rights as property owners and that this use is also trespass, contaminating their land. They seek damages to compensate for a claimed reduction in the market value of their realty and for a personal discomfort, stress, annoyance and anxiety associated with Champion's contamination of the river, the lake, and their personal property. (U.S. District Court East TN Sep. 15, 1992)

Although the plaintiffs testified that damages were incurred because of the pollution, the case was controversial because of the legal restriction. For example, the case had a cutoff date of January 4, 1988, stipulating that any events that happened prior to that date could not be considered. Each side of the case brought toxicologists to discuss their assessment of the dioxin found in the river. Champion's defense team, consisting of an entourage of 25 to 30 lawyers, consultants, paralegals, and secretaries, challenged the information presented by a top expert in the field of toxicology, claiming that dioxin level was non-existent in the fish tissues. But the expert indicated that if there was a discernable level of dioxin, using measures presented by Champion, it would be disastrous. Finally, after 19 futile hours of jury deliberation over five days, the federal judge declared a mistrial.

Champion officials were concerned about publicity from the trial, fearing the likely result of a second trial and the Cocke County residents lacked the funds needed for a second trial. This common concern pushed both sides, Champion and the plaintiffs' lawyers, to seek settlement out of court. Community residents did not agree on the terms which assigned $1.8 million to the landowners' lawyers and only $1,200 for each property owner, as well as releasing Champion from liability for all future claims, demands, or rights of action.

The class action suit filed by the landowners of Cocke County was unprecedented because, after 85 years of pollution, community members as an organized group took the company to court and utilized the legal system. Although the case did not end in the landowners' favor, it does represent another stage of community struggle against pollution.

DISCUSSION

In order to assess the factors that contribute to community responses to chronic technological disaster, this study used multiple methods to provide a broad perspective on such a problem. Historical review of events associated with 85 years of pollution provided different strategies used by a small community to cope with the pollution. Utilizing the Social Process Model (Edelstein, 1988) as a theoretical framework, the study found the history of the pollution to be a significant dimension influencing community responses. The integration of the model enriched the analytical argument in this study. Accordingly, this study generated empirical evidence that supports the Social Process Model propositions.

As the Social Process Model indicated in Postulate 1, toxic exposure involves complex interactions among various levels of society that differ across time and actual dimensions; this study found evidence to support such a proposition. Dealing with the politics of the pollution for over 85 years has caused disappointment and frustration among residents. Failing policies and regulations have caused residents to lose trust in every system that they have relied on to resolve the problem. The most stressful experience that the community has had in the last 15 years is its involvement with the EPA. Community residents interpret the name literally, the *E*nvironmental *P*rotection *A*gency, a federal agency created to ensure protection against hazardous wastes and to protect public safety. But the agency seemed to be a failure to the small community in the mountains. With all the scientific experience and all the laws and regulations, residents have watched the agency lose its credibility because of its inability to enforce the law and its failure to observe the simple reality of a coffee-brown river with an awful smell that can be noticed miles away. Instead, residents believe that the agency was much too involved in scientific jargon and terminologies and that it was actually protecting the polluter's rights (Table 1).

The period between 1980-1993 has been the most critical time in the history of the Pigeon River controversy. During this period, community groups were formed and the fight for a clean river grew to an unprecedented scale. Postulate 2 states that the impacts not only effect how victims behave, but how they perceive and compre-

TABLE 1. Community Trust

Organizational Type	No Trust		Moderate Trust		Great Trust	
	Freq.	%	Freq.	%	Freq.	%
Environmental Action Groups	5	10.2	10	20.4	34	69.4
Scientists & Technologists	9	18	19	39	21	43
Local Government	19	39	16	33	14	29
State Politicians	27	55	15	31	7	14
EPA	37	75.5	8	16	4	8
Champion Int.	47	94	1	2	2	4

*Note: participants expressed their level of trust regarding each organization separately.

hend their lives, in both short and long terms. The survey results show that 86% of the participants believe that the pollution of the river is a very serious matter, while the remaining 14% believe that the pollution is a serious matter and can have long term effects on their lives and on generations to come.

The Pigeon River holds many potential assets for community use, both aesthetically and recreationally. However, the pollution of the river has prevented community residents from drawing upon its resources. An economic impact analysis of the recreational benefits of a restored Pigeon River concluded that, if cleaned, it has prime potential to support recreational activities (Bach & Barnett, 1987). "The recreational activities projected for the Pigeon River can be subdivided into the following activities: (1) commercial raft floating; (2) other watercraft sport (canoes, kayaks); (3) fishing; and (4) other general recreation" (p. 7). From the period 1988 through 1997, the projected total direct benefits derived from recreational use of a clean Pigeon River are $18,332,803, which averages $1,833,280 per year. The total economic impact equals $73,331,212, which averages $7,333,121 per year.

Assessing the missed economic benefits from recreational activities alone, residents believe that the pollution of the Pigeon River is an economic disaster with long-lasting impacts. Aside from the expected increase in revenue if the river was clean, job opportunities would be enhanced and industrial investments would increase. In 1989, Cocke County's per capita income was $8,574, in comparison to the State of Tennessee's per capita income of $12,255 (U.S. Bureau of Census, 1988). Such economic impacts are caused by the conditions of the Pigeon River, where most of the county residents believe that the pollution has deprived the community of economic development and constituted a barrier for industrial development.

Stressful effects caused by exposure to toxic materials was addressed in Postulate 3, 'toxic exposure incidents are stressful, forcing victims to adopt some form of coping responses'. Stress was found to be dominant among community residents. Based on the results of the structured interviews, over 80% of the respondents exhibited qualitative stress, scored using the observational and coding techniques mentioned earlier based on the four parameters: level of family agreement, tone of voice, anger, and frustration. Family members expressed feelings of worthlessness, powerlessness and despair regarding the condition of the river.

Coping with a disaster of this magnitude is assumed to vary based on people's abilities and resources. The Social Process Model indicates that coping patterns may vary across time. This postulate is also verified in particular through the examination and presentation of multiple coping responses that have been adopted by a small isolated community lacking essential resources.

Community members may have participated in at least one of the three coping strategies addressed earlier. Being in a situation that has prevailed for years and receiving no actual help from political organizations have produced many negative feelings among community residents toward the outside world. Community members raised complaints to every level. However, the responses were politicized. This atmosphere was obvious to community residents over the years and was inherited from generation to generation. People from the Cocke County community exhibit a sense of fear of the powerful opponent that has succeeded for 85 years in manipulating the process and challenging the community's will to improve the river's conditions. This sense of fear has been transformed into feelings of apathy among some community members. Participation in organized community actions (i.e., holding meetings, signing petitions, educating the public, and raising funds) is considered one of the coping strategies which has helped community members foster their anger and frustration.

Finally, Postulate 4 indicates that contamination is inherently stigmatizing and arouses anticipatory fears. In Cocke County, residents have been aware of the risk associated with the pollution of the river particularly since the discovery of dioxin. Health fears emerged after a number of residents who lived close to the river contracted and died of cancer. After almost 90 years of pollution, residents believe that Champion has exceeded all decent societal norms and ethics and the company's quest for profit has led to actions that are immoral. Most residents believe that, because of the contaminated river, new investors have not been encouraged to open businesses in the community. Evidence indicated that the farming industry lost contracts with Bush Canning due to the belief that farmers used water from the contaminated Pigeon River for irrigation. Improving the condition of the river seems to be impossible to a majority of residents who believe nothing will change "because Champion has the power and the money."

Considering the Social Process Model, this study shows the complexity of chronic technological disaster and its effect on multiple levels in the community, including political, economic and cultural aspects.

IMPLICATIONS FOR SOCIAL WELFARE PRACTICE

Evidence showed that chronic technological disaster may have multiple impacts on rural communities as predicted by the Social Process Model. In terms of responses to this type of disaster, rural communities tend to lack the necessary resources to fight the disaster. The historical review of the Pigeon River problem indicates that community action seems to be the most effective method. However, for a small community with limited resources, many challenges must be considered.

Although the community struggled without any apparent help from a social worker, their efforts might have been more fruitful much earlier, had they been guided by one. For instance, through the help of a social worker, residents who have developed apathy and fear over the years may have been encouraged to become active in the fight against the pollution of the Pigeon River. The ultimate goal of a social worker's involvement is to promote awareness among community members in order to bring about necessary change. A social worker who possesses knowledge, skills and experience in community organization may be a great help to contaminated communities in advocating and promoting empowerment and self-enhancement. Social workers may be active in the process of community change by performing a variety of roles in this process, including initiator, negotiator, advocate, spokesperson, organizer, mediator, and consultant (Kirst-Ashman & Hull, 1995). These macro skills are central to social work practice in communities and can be helpful in assisting communities that are impacted by this type of pollution.

The findings of this case study support recommendations in macro practice interventions such as community actions. Social welfare practitioners should be aware of the multiple dimensions involved with exposure to toxic materials. Comprehensive understanding of the impacts of toxic exposure on the individual, the family and the community is crucial for social work intervention.

In terms of implications for research, more studies are needed to assess the impact of environmental disaster on rural and small communities. Future research might be helpful in determining the relationship between poverty and exposure to toxic waste. Based on this study, the multiple impacts of toxic waste should be considered in the context of community development and change. Further research might be helpful in determining the impact of the historical dimension on the process of toxic exposure.

REFERENCES

Bach, O., and Barnett, W. (1987) *An Economic Impact Analysis on the Recreational Benefits of a Restored Pigeon River.* Walters State Community College, Tennessee.

Bachrach, K., and Zautra, A. (1985) Coping with a community stressor: The threat of a hazardous waste facility. *Journal of Health and Social Behavior.* 26, 127-141.

Boss, P. (1987). Family Stress. In M. Sussman, & S. Steinmets (Eds.). *Handbook of Marriage and the Family.* New York: Plenum Press.

Chess, W., & Norlin, J. (1991). *Human Behavior and the Social Environment: A Social System Model*. Massachusetts: Allyn and Bacon.

Copeland, A., & White, K. (1991). *Studying Families*. Newbury Park: Sage.

Edelstein, M. (1988) *Contaminated Communities–The Social and Psychological Impacts of Residential Toxic Exposure*. Boulder: Westview Press.

Epstein, S., Brown, L., and Pope, C. (1982) *Hazardous Waste in America*. Sierra Club Books, San Francisco.

Erwin, P. (1991). *A Health Assessment of the East Tennessee Region*. Tennessee: Public Health Association, Tennessee.

Kirst-Ashman, K. K., & Hull, G. H. (1995). *Understanding Generalist Practice*. Chicago: Nelson-Hall.

Rogge, M. (1993) Social work, disenfranchised communities, and the natural environment: Field education opportunities. *Journal of Social Work Education*. 29 (1) 111-120.

Schacher, W. (1992) Assessment of water quality, aquatic plants benthic and fisheries. Communities of the Pigeon River, Cocke County, TN. Aquatic Habitat Protection Project TWRA, Region IV.

Tennessee Department of Employment Security. (1993). *Annualized Unemployment Rates–Not Seasonally Adjusted*. March, 1993.

Tennessee Valley Authority. (1983). Champion International Corporation's Effluent Discharge Data for Flow, Color, and Dissolved Solids (1978-1983) as Compiled by the Tennessee Valley Authority.

The Plain Talk. (1912). Local Newspaper Cocke County, Tennessee.

The Plain Talk. (1923). Local Newspaper Cocke County, Tennessee.

U.S. Bureau of the Census. (1988). *County and City Data Book*. Washington.

Social Vulnerability to Toxic Risk

Mary E. Rogge

SUMMARY. A model of social vulnerability to toxic risk from fugitive chemical releases is tested in 8 southeastern U.S. states. Using structural equation modeling techniques, population density emerged as the critical factor driving exposure to toxic risk. Results indicate that: social vulnerability varies across types and sources of toxic risk; social factors, such as race, that increase risk in some circumstances may buffer risk in others; and that toxic risk has both social *justice* and social *welfare* components. Practice and research implications include the importance of community planning and economic models that enhance environmental quality and health along with economic security. *[Article copies available for a fee from The Haworth Document Delivery Service: 1-800-342-9678. E-mail address: getinfo@haworth.com]*

Studies show that higher percentages of minorities and less wealth in communities are related to greater risk of exposure to pollution and toxic waste (United Church of Christ [UCC], 1987; Mohai & Bryant, 1992). Martin-Brown (1992) captures the essence of the inequitable distribution of exposure to toxic substances in her

Mary E. Rogge is Instructor at the College of Social Work, University of Tennessee-Knoxville, 225 Henson Hall, Knoxville, TN 39776, and doctoral candidate at George Warren Brown School of Social Work, Washington University in St. Louis.

The author thanks Dr. David Gillespie of Washington University, Dr. John Orme, Dr. Terri Combs-Orme and the co-editors of this volume for their helpful comments on earlier drafts of this paper.

[Haworth co-indexing entry note]: "Social Vulnerability to Toxic Risk." Rogge, Mary E. Co-published simultaneously in *Journal of Social Service Research* (The Haworth Press, Inc.) Vol. 22, No. 1/2, 1996, pp. 109-129; and: *Research on Social Work and Disasters* (ed: Calvin L. Streeter and Susan A. Murty) The Haworth Press, Inc., 1996, pp. 109-129. Single or multiple copies of this article are available for a fee from The Haworth Document Delivery Service [1-800-342-9678, 9:00 a.m. - 5:00 p.m. (EST). E-mail address: getinfo@haworth.com].

statement that these are places where "disposable waste" is dumped among "disposable people" to generate "disposable income" for others.

The research described in this article expands the analysis of factors associated with disposable, socially vulnerable communities to include factors other than race and economic resources. A model of social vulnerability to toxic risk is tested which hypothesizes that social, economic, demographic and political factors work together to create conditions of social vulnerability to toxic exposure. Structural equation modeling techniques are used to provide a more rigorous test of the relationships between social, demographic and economic factors and toxic risk than has been used in previous studies.

LITERATURE AND THEORETICAL BACKGROUND

Social work has traditionally sought to reduce risk and harm from social problems affecting vulnerable populations in society. Since the professionalization of social work in the early 1900s, social workers have worked to reduce poverty and improve the living conditions of poor and working class citizens through sanitary, safe, healthy housing and work environment (Piven & Cloward, 1977; Pumphrey & Pumphrey, 1961). Of particular concern early on were the harmful effects of crowded, dirty, unsanitary environments on infant mortality and children's wellbeing (Trattner, 1974). Although concerns about the quality of the physical environment are rooted historically in social work, the profession's involvement with the social problems embedded in technological and natural hazards has been limited (Gillespie et al., 1993; Khinduka, 1977). However, there is a growing literature that illuminates the risk to communities from exposure to environmental and technological hazards, including toxic chemicals (Hoff & McNutt, 1994). For social service practitioners, distinguishing between the *social welfare* effects of toxic exposure and *social justice* effects provides a useful framework for assessing and ameliorating toxic risk in communities (Rogge, 1994). For any community exposed to toxic chemicals through industrial releases or toxic waste sites, there is a threat to the social welfare of citizens through harm to physical health, mental health, and economic well-being. Social justice for "disposable" communities at greater risk for toxic exposure is a key call to action for social workers, as was the call to action of the War on Poverty.

The construct of social vulnerability to toxic risk used in this study is derived from research on toxic exposure and epidemiological research. The relationship between race and toxic risk has been a focal point for both empirical research and social action (Bullard, 1990). Evidence that higher percentages of minority populations predicted the distribution of toxic waste has been found in studies of communities at county and city levels (U.S. General Accounting Office, 1983), and at the zip code level of analysis (Gould and Council of Economic Priorities, 1986; UCC, 1987). Hamilton (1993) found that higher proportions of minority populations at the county level predicted decisions by commercial hazardous waste facilities to maintain their capacity, but not to expand. Anderton et al. (1994), however, did not find this relationship at the census tract level. Low income, low household values, and greater proportions of non-white and elderly citizens increase the likelihood of having toxic waste sites in a community (Greenburg & Anderson, 1984; Been, 1994). This mixed empirical evidence demands further research to specify the relationship between minority populations and toxic risk.

Epidemiological studies suggest that social, demographic, and economic characteristics differentiate vulnerability to diseases that are causally related to toxic exposure. Goldman (1991), for example, found race, income and asset levels, family structure, marital status, education, population density, and geographic location to be associated with mortality rates from heart disease, birth defects, and some types of cancer. Aday (1993) identified these characteristics, as well as age, gender, quality of housing and employment type as indicators of physical, mental, and social health in the United States. It is difficult to clearly establish a causal link between mortality and morbidity rates and specific sources of toxic exposure because of the lack of knowledge about the effects of individual chemicals, multiple sources of chemical exposure and risk, associations of personal risk behavior such as smoking with poor health, inadequate measurement technology, and, at times, institutional efforts to obfuscate data for fear of lawsuits or negative repercussions (Wynne, 1987). For these reasons, it is important to note that this study examines the risk, or probability of exposure, to toxic chemicals, rather than actual exposure, or person-chemical contact.

Theoretical Foundation. The conceptualization of social vulnerability and toxic risk draws primarily from distributive justice theory, which defines mechanisms for the fair exchange and allocation of public goods and bads (Cook & Hegtvedt, 1983). The predominant distributive justice theory in the United States can be described as market justice (Tool, 1983) in which the distribution of public goods is determined by unconstrained "natural" economic processes. According to market justice, the worth and significance of actors are demonstrated by their relative market share of income. Citizens who produce lower shares of the market, such as certain minorities, are valued less because they have relatively little to share. In this way, economic worth becomes firmly linked with particular social or racial characteristics. These characteristics indicate social vulnerability, a construct that determines how much people are at risk by virtue of the degree to which they are valued in the market. This traditional form of economic logic is antithetical to perspectives of social justice in which individuals have inherent worth regardless of economic status. According to market justice, and contrary to social work's value base, it is fair and just to deposit public bads, including sources of toxic risk, in socially vulnerable communities because they contribute little to the market economy. Under market justice, these communities are disposable (Martin-Brown, 1992).

MODEL AND HYPOTHESES

The study examines the research question: do county-level, aggregate population characteristics predict social vulnerability to toxic risk? Social vulnerability is conceptualized as a continuum in which lower levels of a social resource, such as education or income, increase social vulnerability, and higher levels decrease it. The theory of social vulnerability to toxic risk is assessed using county-level data in a multi-sample path analysis. Because of the centrality of racial discrimination in studies about toxic waste sites, and indications that race moderates toxic risk, the model is tested in split samples of counties based on racial composition.

Each of the social vulnerability indicators, with the exception of the proportion of citizens voting, is hypothesized to have direct and indirect influences on toxic risk (Figure 1). In counties where social vulnerability is greater, facilities are hypothesized to pollute more because they have fewer institutional constraints and fewer negative consequences for doing so. Greater population density is hypothesized to directly increase toxic risk. Higher proportions of college-educated citizens, age-independent populations, proportion of the population owning their own homes, median income, and proportion of citizens voting indicate less vulnerability and are expected to directly decrease toxic risk. With the exception of the negative hypothesized effect of population density on citizen voting (greater concentrations of people reduce a sense of personal commitment to a community, resulting in proportionally less voting), the positive indirect pathways suggest that the social resources in earlier stages of the model contribute to the accumulation of greater social resources at later stages. Median income and the proportion of home ownership increase as the educated wage-earner pool increases. Each of these social resources increases citizens' freedom and motivation to vote. And, as Hamilton (1993) suggests, greater capacity for collective action, as measured through political participation, reduces toxic risk as firms seek to avoid opposition to their pollution-producing activities.

MEASUREMENT

Toxic risk is measured by the *density (pounds/square mile) of fugitive chemical releases*. Fugitive releases are emissions of particles or gases emitted to the air through parts of facilities other than airstacks, such as pumps or valves. The data are drawn from the EPA's 1992 Toxic Release Inventory (TRI).[1] Since 1987, 20 types of industrial and commercial manufacturing facilities, including chemicals and petroleum, rubber and plastic, textiles, lumber, paper and printing facilities, are required to report yearly their manufacture, use or storage of 313 toxic chemicals. TRI chemicals range in known potency and effect, including, for example, the carcinogen and mutagen ethylene oxide, used to fumigate medical instruments and spices, and to make automotive antifreeze and polyester (Harte et al., 1991). TRI data are not weighted by chemical potency; this study uses aggregate pounds of chemicals released as an overall indicator of risk. By using chemical releases as the source of risk, the generalizability of research that has focused on toxic waste sites as the source of risk is examined.

Population density, age independence, college education, percent owner-occupied homes and median household income are measured using 1990 Census data (U.S. Census Bureau, 1990). *Population density* is used as a control of the rural to urban nature of the counties. Stockwell et al. (1993) found that, compared to other social, demographic and economic characteristics, population density was the best indicator of toxic emissions. The hypothesis is that, as county populations grow, demands for services, goods, employment and economic opportunities grow. The number of commercial and industrial facilities that produce, use, and otherwise supply the

FIGURE 1. Hypothesized Model of Social Vulnerability and Toxic Risk

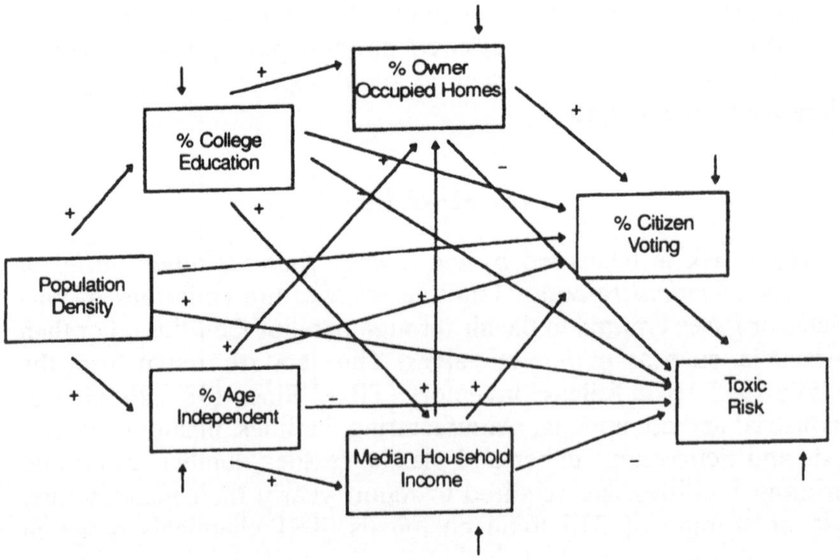

services and goods increase, with accompanying increases in chemical uses and polluting releases.

Age independency (percent of population between ages 17 and 65) tests the relationship between toxic risk and age-related social vulnerability. Governments and industry have targeted for toxic waste sites neighborhoods where older (age-dependent) citizens live, using the rationale that older citizens have fewer political resources to oppose such sitings (Cerrell Associates, 1984). Although there are no empirical studies of the relationship of young (age-dependent) populations with toxic risk, Wilson (1987) discusses the heightened social vulnerability of communities where higher percentages of children and youth live. Thus, age-dependent youth and elderly are more vulnerable to toxic risk, and age-independent adults are less vulnerable.

As *education*, measured by the percentage of citizens having college degrees, increases, toxic risk decreases. With more education, citizens are better informed of threats from toxic chemicals, better linked to social and occupational networks with which they can organize, and have more problem-solving choices to oppose such threats.

Sherraden's (1991) asset-based social welfare theory describes the distinctive advantages of having fiscal assets such as a home, insurance, or savings in addition to income. This study examines *assets and income*. The higher the median *household income*, the lower is toxic risk. From a market justice perspective, higher income citizens contribute to society and are inappropriate recipients of pollution. Income can purchase legal or political power to oppose local toxic risk and to demand greater compensation for harm. *Household assets* are measured with the percent of owner-occupied homes.[2] In the first national study of race, income, assets, and toxic waste sites (UCC; 1987), the mean owner-occupied home value was a stronger indicator than income of toxic waste site location. Tangible assets and associated intangible assets, such as organizational capital, political capital and access to credit (Sherraden, 1991), constrain chemical facilities from polluting because of potentially high costs from lawsuits, political pressure, and negative public opinion.

The *percentage of citizens voting* in the 1992 presidential election (Scammon & McGillivray, 1993) builds on Hamilton's (1993) finding that the potential for collective action in a county, as measured by these data, was the main factor in commercial toxic waste facility decisions to expand or reduce their waste-processing capacity. When tested with the percent of population voting, median household income, home value, the percent of nonwhite population, and population density were not significant, with the exception that the percent of nonwhite population predicted fewer plans to reduce facility capacity.

The hypothesis that the social vulnerability model works differently based on community *racial composition* is tested with samples split on the percent of African-Americans in the population. Other Census-defined racial groups were too small and lacked enough variance and normality to be analyzed. In the market justice system, discrimination has resulted in people of color, their homes, and their communities being valued less than those of their White counterparts. Insufficient institutional mechanisms for their protection (Wilson, 1987) result in governments and firms locating more polluting facilities in higher minority percentage counties.

METHODS AND ANALYSES

Secondary data from national and regional databases were examined in a cross-sectional comparison of counties. Modeling county-level emissions is reasonable because of imprecise information about dispersal patterns of chemicals released into the air (Stockwell, 1994). Path analyses were performed using the structural equation modeling programs PRELIS 2 and LISREL 8 (Scientific Software International, Inc., 1993) to estimate error terms, assess relations simultaneously, examine multivariate distributions and goodness-of-fit measures, and assess model similarities in a multisample group.

This study examines toxic risk and social vulnerability in the eight southeastern United States that form Region IV of the U.S. Environmental Protection Agency (EPA): Alabama, Georgia, Mississippi, Florida, Kentucky, North and South Carolina, and Tennessee. The South has unique cultural, historical, political, and economic development elements; the southern states share a history of slavery in a rural agricultural and plantation economy, defeat in the Civil War, and a long-standing conservative one-party political system (Key, 1984). In recent decades, the region is experiencing a significant shift in urbanization and an industrial and service economy base (Grantham, 1994).

The sample of 330 counties is derived from the 736 counties in the 8 southeastern states. These counties comprise Region IV of the EPA. This is a convenience sample in that it covers the geographic territory from which the Toxic Release Inventory (TRI) data for the study was derived (Stockwell, 1994). The sampling frame is 23% of the 3,141 counties in the U.S. (Strategic Mapping, Inc., 1993) and 16% of U.S. states. There is no claim of national representativeness because only the southern region of the country is covered.

A multi-stage data cleaning and reduction process resulted in the final sample of 330 counties. There are no missing values for the variables used in this study. The sample size was first reduced by removing 175 counties that had no chemical releases. Second, transformations and case elimination through univariate and multivariate diagnostics using LISREL greatly improved but did not reach multivariate normality. LISREL provides more information about the multi-normality of the data, allowing more stringent application of methods such as case elimination to normalize the data (Bollen, 1989). Two hundred and forty counties were removed as univariate and multivariate outliers and extremes that compromised sample representativeness. Case elimination was stopped when no further extreme cases were identified through multiple regression diagnostics.[3] Multivariate skewness with the 330 counties was 7.945 (z-score) at p. = 0.00; multivariate kurtosis was -2.328 at p. = 0.01; χ^2 was 68.534 (p. = 0.00). The model was estimated with generalized least squares (GLS), appropriate for moderately non-normal distributions, rather than maximum likelihood, which assumes multi-normal distributions (Joreskog & Sorbom, 1993). The final sample size of 330 counties is sufficient for analysis, using the criteria of 10-15 cases per independent variable (Tanaka, 1992). No curvilinear relations or interactions were found within the model. Table 1 shows means, standard deviations, and covariance matrix.

TABLE 1. Means, Standard Deviations, and Covariance Matrix (n = 330)

	Pop. D.	% Age	% Educ	Md. Inc	% Home	% Vote	Fug. R
Population Density	**0.06**						
% Age Independent	0.44	**7.44**					
% College Education	0.02	0.15	**0.02**				
Median Income	0.01	0.16	0.01	**0.01**			
% Owner-Occ. Homes	−0.36	0.49	−0.29	−0.02	**27.96**		
% Citizens Voting	−0.41	−2.63	0.02	−0.04	9.78	**40.16**	
Fugitive Release Density	0.03	0.20	0.01	0.01	−0.14	−0.04	**0.03**
Mean	(64.23[1])	59.77	(13.49)	(21,901)	66.5	51.66	(105.61)
	.922		**1.13**	**4.34**			**.914**
S.D.	**.24**[2]	2.73	**.14**	**.08**	5.29	6.34	**.186**

1 Figure in ( ) is raw data equivalent of transformed variable; transformed value is **boldfaced.**
2 Transformed value is **boldfaced.**

PATH STRUCTURE AND RELATIONSHIPS

The social vulnerability indicators together (Figure 2) accounted for 61% of the variance in fugitive release density ($R^2 = .61$, $t = 12.81$). Goodness-of-fit measures indicate the model fits the data (Joreskog, 1993): $\chi^2 = 2.07$ (p. = .72), df = 4, the root mean square error of approximation (RMSEA) is 0.0, with RMSEA confidence intervals (c.i.) of 0.0 - 0.061. The largest standardized residual is −1.22.

Table 2 shows the decomposition of direct, indirect and total effects of each indicator on fugitive release density. Each indicator has significant direct effects. As hypothesized, population density increases toxic risk, while household income and age independency mitigate it. Contrary to hypothesized relations, higher levels of home ownership, education and citizen voting are positively linked with toxic risk. Higher levels of these indicators, typically considered buffers from harm in studies of toxic waste sites, increase the risk of harm from toxic chemical releases.

Population density has by far the strongest total effect (Beta = .74; t = 19.84). In fact, a regression run with only population density accounts for 54% of the variance explained ($\chi^2 = .021$; df = 1; RMSEA = 0.0; RMSEA c.i = 0.0 -0.072). The 7% variance added to the model by the other indicators is not significant (χ^2 difference =

FIGURE 2. Social Vulnerability and Fugitive Release Density (n = 330)

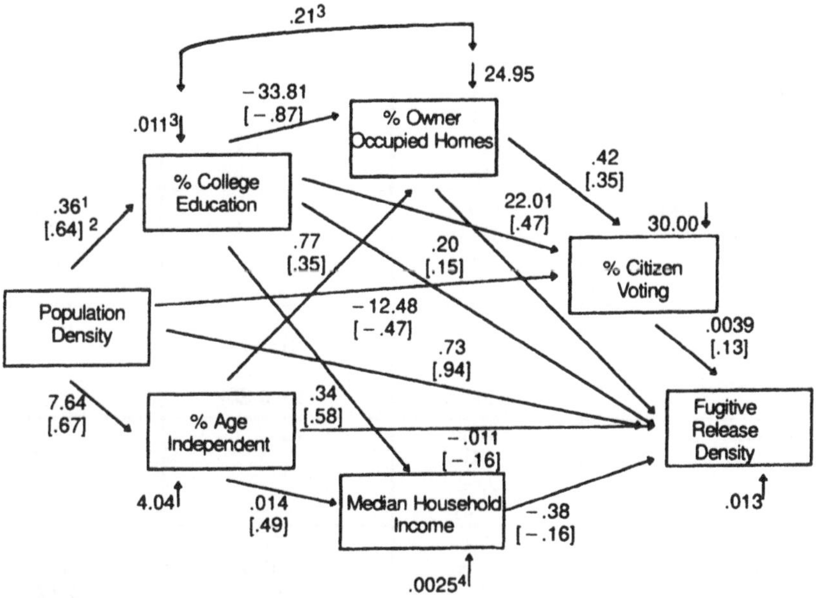

Model R^2 = .61
error variance: .013 (.0011) 12.81
χ^2 = 2.07 (p = .72), df = 4
RMSEA = 0.0; RMSEA 90% confidence intervals (0.0 - 0.061)
1 unstandardized beta coefficient
2 standardized Beta
3 standardized Betas for error terms and correlated error terms not reported in LISREL
all reported coefficients are significant at p $\leq$ .01
4 error terms of household income and education are correlated .00

2.047, df difference = 3, p. = .58). Consistent with Stockwell et al.'s (1993) findings, toxic risk from industrial and commercial chemical releases is primarily driven upward by growing population pressure.

Age independency, income, home ownership, and voting have weak total effects on toxic risk; education has no significant effect. Age independency (total Beta = −0.17) and income (total Beta = −0.16) have small mitigating effects. This suggests that higher income levels and proportions of age independent adults (relative to children and the elderly) exert a dampening influence on toxic risk in more densely populated areas. As expected, the voting popula-

TABLE 2. Total, Direct and Indirect Effects of Social Vulnerability Characteristics on Fugitive Density (n = 330)

Variable	Direct	Indirect[1]	Total
Population density	0.73[2] (.046)[3] 15.79[4] **[.94]**[5]	−0.16 (0.04) −4.04 **[−0.20]**	0.57 (0.03) 19.84 **[0.74]**
Age dependency	−0.011 (.0038) −2.81 **[−.16]**	ns	−0.01 (0.00) −3.47 **[−0.17]**
College	0.20 (.075) 2.72 **[.15]**	−0.28 (0.08) −3.30 **[−0.20]**	ns
Income	−0.38 (0.14) −2.66 **[−.16]**	ns	−0.38 (0.14) −2.64 **[−0.16]**
% Owner-occupied homes	.0052 (.0015) 3.41 **[.15]**	0.00 (0.00) 2.97 **[0.05]**	0.01 (0.00) 4.77 **[0.20]**
Citizen voting	.0039 (.0012) 3.32 **[.13]**	- - - - -	0.00 (0.00) 3.32 **[0.13]**

1 the total indirect effect is the aggregate indirect effect through all significant paths.
2 unstandardized b coefficient
3 standard error of the parameter estimate
4 t-value
5 standardized Beta regression coefficient
all reported coefficients are significant at $p \leq .01$

tion decreases as population density increases, however, the small positive association between voting and toxic risk is unexpected. One explanation is that citizens are politically active to maintain and enhance economic development. Similar to logging communities in the northwestern United States, faced with the threat of losing either economic security or degrading environmental resources, toxic risk may be a lower priority, or no priority.

The endogenous indicators do not add significantly to the model, therefore their indirect effects will not be decomposed. However, the relationships suggest a picture of the population in these counties. The indirect paths are as hypothesized, with interesting exceptions. First, income is not related to home-ownership or voting, indicating that patterns of home-ownership and voting are similar across income levels. Second, the combination of less education with greater home-ownership, and more home-ownership with less income, suggests working class citizens. Third, the missing link between age independence and voting suggests that the potential for collective political action depends on factors other than a critical mass of actors.

Because of the singular importance of population density, the most important indirect effects are those of population density on toxic risk through the endogenous indicators. The lack of significant variance added by these indicators suggests the contribution here to be small, yet instructive for future study. The key finding here (Table 2) is that some social vulnerability indicators (−.20) mitigate population density's very strong direct effect (.94). Examination of the indirect paths shows the mitigation is in the linkage of population density, education, age-dependency, and income. These relationships can be summarized by reporting the standardized total Beta coefficients ($p. \leq .01$) of population density on these indicators: education (.64), age-independency (.67), and income (.70). These moderate positive relationships strengthen the mitigating effects of income and age-independency on toxic risk.

Two sets of correlated error terms indicate specification error in the model. The error terms of median household income and education (.00, $t = 4.32$), and of education and percent of owner-occupied homes (.21, $t = 4.51$) are correlated. The correlated errors suggest that these measures of economic resources and human capital are components of a larger construct of economic assets and human capital.

The overall picture of southern counties facing greater toxic risk from chemical emissions is of urban, working class counties. Toxic risk is greater where the proportion of potential wage-earning adults is smaller, and the proportion of children and elderly are higher. Working class citizens are more likely to live and work where industrial and commercial enterprises, that support a full range of daily community living, are located. Toxic risk increases with citizen voting, an indicator of political action. Rather than assume that citizens are voting for more pollution, citizen participation is more likely tied to a higher level of economic activity and search for economic security, which is linked to greater demand for more diverse services and goods, which is linked to the production of chemical releases as by-products of meeting the demand.

The cadres of working class adults in these counties are likely to be concerned about maintaining jobs and enhancing economic opportunities. If toxic risk is perceived as a threat, it is likely to be a lower priority than economic security. A belief in traditional modes of economic development, in conjunction with relatively recent economic expansion in the South, are likely to result in a lack of attention, or opposition to, environmental regulations that could reduce toxic risk (Grantham, 1994; Bullard, 1990).

Racial Composition Split Samples. To examine if the model operates differently in different racial communities, the 330 counties were split using the "tipping point" (perception that people of color attain equal or majority status when their actual proportion reaches 30%; see Davis & Proctor, 1989). Counties in the low percent African-American group (n = 218) have less than 30% African-Americans; the high group (n = 112) has 30% or more. Descriptive statistics (Table 3) suggest that southern, predominantly White counties have significantly higher toxic risk (169%), population density (155%), and higher proportions of income (114%), age independent adults (104%) and home ownership (104%). Voting and education are similar in their effect. Contrary to studies showing minority communities to be more vulnerable to toxic risk, this bivariate data suggests that predominantly African-American counties, although economically and geographically more isolated, poorer in income and assets, and having higher proportions of children and elderly, are less socially vulnerable to toxic risk. The distinction appears to be the difference in the source and type of toxic risk. Previous studies showing high degrees of association between minority status and toxic risk have concentrated on toxic waste sites as the source of risk, whereas this study examines toxic chemical releases. The implications are at least threefold: (1) social vulnerability to toxic risk is not necessarily generalizable across types and sources of toxic risk; (2) social factors that increase risk

TABLE 3. Social Vulnerability and Toxic Risk Characteristics: Low and High African-American Groups

	Low Minority (n = 218)		High Minority (n = 122)	
	Mean	(S.D.)	Mean	(S.D.)
Pop Density[1]	72.90	(0.222)	46.94	(0.245)
Age Indep[1]	60.68	(2.297)	58.12	(2.649)
% College	13.24	(0.145)	13.69	(0.117)
% Home Own[1]	67.43	(4.955)	64.67	(5.459)
Med Income[1]	$22,682.00	(0.077)	$19,858.00	(0.072)
% Voting	52.13	(5.905)	50.75	(7.043)
Fugitive Release[1] Density	117.33	(0.183)	69.24	(0.186)

1 p < .01

in some circumstances may buffer risk in others; and (3) both the social justice and social welfare components of toxic risk must be attended to.

Multivariate normality was not attained for the multi-sample path analysis of the two groups. For the low percent African-American group, the standardized z-score was 7.161 (p. = 0.00), standardized kurtosis was −1.438 (p. = 0.075), χ^2 was 53.351 (p. = 0.00). For the high percent African-American group, the standardized z-score was 7.440 (p. = 0.00), standardized kurtosis was −0.928 (p. = 0.177), and χ^2 was 56.222 (p. = 0.00). GLS was used to estimate the model. Goodness-of-fit statistics for both models were acceptable. For the low percent African-American group, .58% of the variance was explained, with a χ^2 of 8.16 (p. = .52), df = 9, RMSEA = 0, RMSEA c.i. = 0.0-7.2. For the high percent African-American group, 65% of the variance was explained, with a χ^2 of 12.51 (p. = .57), df = 14, RMSEA = 0.0, RMSEA c.i. = 0.0 - .083. The error covariance between education and percent of owner-occupied homes retained significance in both groups.

The multi-sample comparison using LISREL showed the path model structures, path coefficients, error covariances, and error variances of the two groups to be different; however, the 7% greater variance (.R^2 = .58, .65) explained in the high percent African-American group was not significant (χ^2 difference = 4.35; df difference = 5.0, p. = .50; Pagano, 1986). As with the non-split sample of 330 counties, the variance added by the endogenous variables was not significant for either racial group: low percent African-American (R^2

population density = .55; R^2 all indicators = .58; χ^2 difference = .8.159; df difference = 8, p. = .40); high percent African-American (R^2 population density = .51; R^2 all indicators = .65; χ^2 difference = 12.51; df difference = 13, p. = .50). Therefore, the dynamics portrayed in the 330 county results best represent the relationships of the social vulnerability indicators to toxic risk from TRI chemicals.

Although the multi-sample models are statistically equivalent to the 330 county model, three differences in particular imply patterns that merit future analysis. First, the overall model accounted for 8% more variance in the high percent African-American counties, and the endogenous indicators within the high percent African-American counties added 14% variance to that of population density compared to 3% in the low percent African-American counties. Future research in which population density is removed from the model and used contextually, as was racial composition in this study, is recommended to understand more specifically how the other social vulnerability indicators operate in communities across a rural-urban continuum. Second, the total mitigating effects of age independency (total effect Beta at $p \leq .01$; high % = .05; low % = $-.38$) is stronger in the high percent African-American counties. This suggests that one strategy to reduce toxic risk in these counties is to increase the proportion of working age individuals. Third, the importance of home ownership and income was quite different in the two models. Income lost significance in the low percent African-American group; home ownership had both direct and indirect positive effects on toxic risk (total effect Beta = .13). In the high percent African-American group, the mitigating effect of income was exclusively through indirect paths (total Beta = $-.17$) and home ownership had only indirect effects (total Beta = .09). These differences, and correlated error terms in the models, point to the need to clarify how assets and income, as two types of economic resources (Sherraden, 1991), influence toxic risk in racially different communities.

CONCLUSIONS

Several conclusions and interventions are suggested by this analysis. First, social vulnerability may differ according to the type and source of toxic risk. Many studies have associated toxic waste sites with the social injustice indicators of race and poverty; this study identified a primary association between toxic chemical releases and the broader, social welfare indicator of population density. Two factors, absent to date from the social vulnerability/toxic risk equation, may be fruitful to examine. Where in the economic/technological production process is the risk located? For example, are toxic chemicals perceived less as a threat during the production process (needed for economic productivity and gain), than at the end-stage of production (used up, waste)? Is it therefore easier to associate end-stage waste with "disposable," vulnerable communities? The second additional factor is the visibility of the risk. While chemical-emitting facilities are no less tangible than toxic waste sites, and visible plumes may be seen at some, many chemical releases are invisible and odorless, providing no cue as to their potential harm (TRI, 1992). Fugitive releases leaking from poorly fit valves and pipes are particularly likely to be invisible. Are, then, community members constrained from conceptualizing chemical releases as a threat, and therefore acting to ameliorate the threat, because it is essentially intangible? Is it, again, easier to locate visible, tangible, identified sources of risk in "disposable" communities?

Second, population density, with an accompanying concentration of commercial and industrial activity, is the single most important indicator of social vulnerability to risk from TRI chemical releases. If greater toxic risk is a given where more people congregate, then we must clarify the actual harm to the population's social welfare–in terms of physical, mental, and economic wellbeing–and work to reduce that harm. The data suggest that interventions be developed simultaneously in urban areas to ameliorate existing toxic risk, and in rural areas to prevent risk as these areas grow (Daly & Cobb, 1989). These findings call for a greater emphasis on coordinating community planning, data on technological hazards, social welfare and justice, and economic development.

Third, the link between social problems and technological hazards such as toxic risk is a clear point of entry for social workers to participate in developing economic models that sustain both people and the environment. More strategies are needed that explicate the link between environmental quality and social welfare, and show that environmental quality need not be sacrificed for economic security (Sagoff, 1988). Whatever the source of toxic risk, particular attention must be paid to strategies for improving economic security that negate discriminatory "market justice" formulations. An economic system in which vulnerable populations are treated as insignificant and disposable is simply, unjustifiably wrong.

An agenda for future research expands the study of social vulnerability and toxic risk spacially, conceptually, and analytically. A best case scenerio is a design that is, first, geographically nested and assesses relationships from census tract to national levels, and second, expands the pool of social vulnerability indicators and compares them across different sources of toxic risk. For example, the effects of additional economic resources and human capital indicators (e.g., employment rates, gender, types of employment, types and ownership of businesses) can be assessed across different sources and types of toxic risk, including TRI data weighted for potency, toxic waste sites, hazardous waste incinerators or pesticide use. Future analyses using population density as a contextual variable to split samples will allow clarification of the relationships suggested in this study, including the effects of social vulnerability indicators in protecting or exacerbating toxic risk and the differential dynamics of income, age independency, assets and income in communities of different racial composition. A third design feature combines increasingly advanced statistical analysis, such as structural equation modeling and latent constructs, with spacial analysis techniques such as mapping with geographic information systems.

Toxic risk is a complicated problem that requires a multi-faceted, multi-disciplinary response. While evidence regarding the social vulnerability dimension of toxic risk is as of yet mixed, it is sufficient to warrant a clear call to action for the social work profession. We must fully participate in efforts to specify and ameliorate the threats to both social welfare and social justice from this by-product of our social affluence.

NOTES

1. The social vulnerability model was assessed using the four types of chemical releases reported in the TRI: releases through facility airstacks, fugitive releases, releases onto land or into water (TRI, 1992), and a combined total release density figure. The model was strongest with fugitive release density [$R^2 = .61$; error variance = .0134 (.0011) 12.81], with twice the variance explained of the next strongest type, airstack density [$R^2 = .30$; error variance = .013 (.038) 12.81]. The model with fugitive density is described here to illustrate the strongest relationships among the variables.

2. A second measure of household assets, the median value of owner-occupied homes, was intercorrelated with median household income. It was examined in a parallel path model, substituting for median household income. The parallel model showed median home value to be a weaker measure than median income. Goodness-of-fit were $\chi^2 = .64$ ($p = .89$), with 3 df, RMSEA = 0.00, RMSEA c.i., 0.00-0.43. Median home value was not significant at $p < .01$ ($b = -.071$, $p = .049$, $t = -1.45$).

3. The stringent approach used here to maximize the multi-normality of the data may influence the path analysis results. Given the resistance of this data to multinormality, the results of this analysis should be compared in the future with other approaches. One alternative, for example, is to use weighted least squares (WLS) to estimate the highly non-normal distributions of the full set of 736 counties.

BIBLIOGRAPHY

Aday, L. (1993). *At Risk in America: The Health and Health Care Needs of Vulnerable Populations in the United States*. San Fransisco, CA: Jossey-Bass.

Anderton, D.L., Anderson, A.B., Rossi, P.H., Oakes, J.M., Fraser, M.R., Weber, E.W., Calabrese, E.J. (1994). Hazardous waste facilities: "Environmental equity" issues in metropolitan areas. *Evaluation Review*. 18(2), 123-140.

Been, V. (1994). Locally undesirable land uses in minority neighborhoods: Disproportionate siting or market dynamics? *Yale Law Journal*. 103(6). 1384-1421.

Bollen, K.A. (1989). *Structural Equations with Latent Variables*. NY: John Wiley & Sons.

Bullard, R.D. (1990). *Dumping in Dixie: Race, Class, and Environmental Quality*. Boulder, CO: Westview Press.

Cerrell Associates (1984). *Political difficulties facing waste to energy conversion plant siting*. Report prepared for the California Waste Management Board.

Cook, K.S. and Hegtvedt, K.A. (1983). Distributive justice, equity, and equality. *Annual Review of Sociology*. 9, 217-241.

Daly, H.E. & Cobb, J.B., Jr. (1989). *For the Common Good: Redirecting the Economy toward Community, the Environment, and a Sustainable Future*. Boston, MA: Beacon Press.

Davis, L.E. & Proctor, E.K. (1989). *Race, Gender and Class: Guidelines for Practice with Individuals, Families, and Groups*. Englewood Cliffs, N.J.: Prentice Hall.

Gillespie, D.F., Colignon, R.A., Banerjee, M.M., Murty, S.A., and Rogge, M.E. (1993). *Partnerships for Community Preparedness*. Boulder, CO: Institute of Behavioral Science, University of Colorado Press.

Goldman, B.A. (1991). *The Truth About Where You Live: An Atlas for Action on Toxins and Mortality*. New York: Random House.

Gould, J. M. and Council of Economic Priorities (1986). *Quality of Life in American Neighborhoods: Levels of Affluence, Toxic Waste, and Cancer Mortality in Residential Zip Code Areas*. Boulder, CO: Westview Press.

Grantham, D.W. (1994). *The South in Modern America: A Region at Odds*. NY: Harper Collins.

Greenburg, M.R. & Anderson, R.F. (1984). *Hazardous Waste Sites: The Credibility Gap*. New Brunswick, N.J.: Center for Urban Policy Research.

Hamilton, J.T. (1993). Politics and social costs: Estimating the impact of collective action on hazardous waste facilities. *RAND Journal of Economics*. (24)1, 101-125.

Harte, J., Holdren, C., Schneider, R., and Shirley, C. (1991). *Toxics a to z: A guide to everyday pollution hazards*. Berkeley, CA: University of California Press.

Hoff, M.D. & McNutt,. J.G. (1994). *The Global Environmental Crisis: Implications for Social Welfare and Social Work*. Aldershot, England: Avebury.

Joreskog, K.G. (1993). Testing Structural Equation Models. In K.A. Bollen and J.S. Long (Eds.) *Testing Structural Equation Models*. (294-316). Newbury Park, CA: Sage.

Joreskog, K.G. & Sorbom, D. (1993). *LISREL: Structural Equation Modeling with the SIMPLIS Command Language*. Hillsdale, N.J.: Lawrence Erlbaum Associates.

Key, V.O. (1984). *Southern Politics in State and Nation*. Knoxville, TN: University of Tennessee Press.

Khinduka, S.K. (1977). *Environments, People and Places: Social Work Education and Human Settlements*. International Association of Schools of Social Work, Annual Conference Proceedings. 36-50.

Martin-Brown, J. & Ofosu-Amaah, W. (1992). *Proceedings of the global assembly of women and the environment: Partners in life*. Washington, DC: United Nations Environmental Programme and World WIDE Network, Inc.

Mohai, P. & Bryant, B. (1992). *Environmental Racism: Reviewing the Evidence*. Draft, Paper presented at the University of Michigan Law School Symposium on Race, Poverty, and the Environment, January 23, 1992.

Pagano, R.R. (1986). *Understanding Statistics in the Behavioral Sciences*. New York: West.

Piven, F. & Cloward, R. (1977). *Poor People's Movements*. New York: Pantheon Books.

Pumphrey, R.E. & Pumphrey, M.W. (1961). *The Heritage of American Social Work: Readings in its Philosophical and Institutional Development*. New York: Columbia University Press.

Rogge, M.E. (1994). Environmental injustice: Social welfare and toxic waste. In M.D. Hoff, & J.G. McNutt. (Eds.). (1994). *The Global Environmental Crisis:*

Implications for Social Welfare and Social Work. (53-74). Aldershot, England: Avebury.

Sagoff, M. (1989). *The Economy of the Earth: Philosophy, Law, and the Environment*. New York: Cambridge University Press.

Scammon, R.M. & McGillivray, A.V. (Eds.). (1993). *American Votes: A Handbook of Contemporary American Election Statistics*. Washington, DC: Election Research Center, Congressional Quarterly.

Scientific Software International, Inc. (1993). *LISREL and PRELIS for Windows*. Chicago, IL: Scientific Software International, Inc.

Sherraden, M. (1991). *Assets and the Poor: A New American Welfare Policy*. Armonk, New York: M.E. Sharpe.

Stockwell, J.R. (1994). U.S. EPA Region IV. 345 Courtland Street, N.E. Atlanta, GA.Waste Management Division, Federal Facilities Branch. Personal Communication, May 12, June 10-14, 1994.

Stockwell, J.R., Sorenson, J.W., Eckert, J.W., Jr. & Carreras, E.M. (1993). The U.S. EPA geographic information system for mapping environmental releases of toxic chemical release inventory (TRI) chemicals. *Risk Analysis*. 13(2). 155-164.

Strategic Mapping, Inc. (1993). *Atlas GIS Command Reference*. Santa Fe, CA: Strategic Mapping, Inc.

Tanaka, J.S. (1993). Multifaceted conceptions of fit in structural equation models. In K.A. Bollen and J.S. Long (Eds.) *Testing Structural Equation Models*. (10-39). Newbury Park, CA: Sage.

Tool, M.R. (1983). Equational justice and social value. *Journal of Economic Issues*. 17:2, 335-344.

Toxic Release Inventory (1992). *Toxic Release Inventory CD-ROM Technical Documentation*. CD-ROM. Washington, DC: U.S. Environmental Protection Agency.

Trattner, W. I. (1974). *From Poor Law to Welfare State: A History of Social Welfare in America*. New York: Free Press.

U.S. Census Bureau (1990). Census of Population and Housing, 1990. Summary Tape File 1. Washington, DC: U.S. Bureau of the Census.

U.S. General Accounting Office (June, 1983). *Siting of Hazardous Waste Landfills and Their Correlation with the Racial and Socio-economic Status of Surrounding Communities*. Report No. GAO/RCED-83-168. Washington, DC: United States Government Printing Office.

United Church of Christ, Commission for Racial Justice (1987). *Toxic Wastes and Race in the United States: A National Report on the Racial and Socio-economic Characteristics of Communities with Hazardous Waste Sites*. United Church of Christ, Commission for Racial Justice, New York.

Wilson, W.J. (1987). *The Truly Disadvantaged: The Inner City, the Underclass, and Public Policy*. Chicago: University of Chicago Press.

Wynne, B. (1987). Hazardous waste: What kind of issue? in B. Wynne (Ed.). *Risk Management and Hazardous Waste: Implementation and the Dialectics of Credibility*, Springer-Verlag, New York, pp. 45-83.

Inter-Agency Collaboration and Hazards Education in American Communities

Charles E. Faupel
Jack Kartez

SUMMARY. There is a growing literature on hazards education and its effectiveness in prompting appropriate mitigation, preparedness

---

Charles E. Faupel is Professor in the Department of Sociology at Auburn University. He has been involved in disaster research for more than 15 years and has authored two books in the area: *Disaster Beliefs and Emergency Planning* (with Dennis Wenger and Thomas James), and *The Ecology of Disaster*. Dr. Faupel has also published articles on disaster and the environment in several journals, including *Human Organization*, *Sociological Spectrum*, *International Journal of Mass Emergencies and Disasters*, *Society and Natural Resources*, and *Environment and Behavior*, among others. Jack Kartez is Director of the Environmental Science and Policy Program at the University of Southern Maine. His hazards-related research has received support from the National Science Foundation, the U.S. Environmental Protection Agency, and nongovernmental organizations. Dr. Kartez has published on environmental hazards in numerous journals including the *Journal of the American Planning Association*, *Environmental Management*, *Industrial Crisis Quarterly*, *Disasters*, and *Environmental Impact Assessment Review*.

The authors are especially grateful to David Gillespie for his helpful comments on an earlier draft of this paper. This research was supported in part by Grant #BCS 92-03385 from the National Science Foundation. Revision of a paper read at the Annual Meetings of the Mid-South Sociological Association, Lafayette, LA, October, 1994. Opinions expressed are solely those of the authors and do not necessarily reflect the position of the National Science Foundation.

[Haworth co-indexing entry note]: "Inter-Agency Collaboration and Hazards Education in American Communities." Faupel, Charles E. and Jack Kartez. Co-published simultaneously in *Journal of Social Service Research* (The Haworth Press, Inc.) Vol. 22, No. 1/2, 1996, pp. 131-149; and: *Research on Social Work and Disasters* (ed: Calvin L. Streeter and Susan A. Murty) The Haworth Press, Inc., 1996, pp. 131-149. Single or multiple copies of this article are available for a fee from The Haworth Document Delivery Service [1-800-342-9678, 9:00 a.m. - 5:00 p.m. (EST). E-mail address: getinfo@haworth.com].

and response activities on the part of individuals and families. There has been virtually nothing written, however, on what factors tend to account for such hazards education activities in the first place. Factors that may account for varying levels of hazards education activities, such as prior disaster experience, hazards risk, and coordination between emergency management and planning offices, are examined in three separate multiple regression analyses. Generally, we found that (1) the *frequency of engaging in oral and written hazards education activities* is significantly affected only by the level of preparedness activities on the part of emergency managers that involve some sort of exchange with other city agencies; (2) the *frequency of conducting hazards education workshops* is affected by the level of inter-agency preparedness efforts (above), the breadth of hazards risks confronted by a community, and by the frequency of interaction between emergency managers and city planners; and (3) the *breadth of hazards education audiences* is also significantly affected by the level of interagency preparedness efforts, the breadth of hazards risks, and the frequency of interaction between emergency managers and city planners. Policy implications, particularly as they relate to social service delivery organizations, are also discussed. *[Article copies available for a fee from The Haworth Document Delivery Service: 1-800-342-9678. E-mail address: getinfo@haworth.com]*

INTRODUCTION

There is an emerging literature on hazards education which has focused primarily on either (1) documenting the level of hazards awareness and knowledge among populations in the United States; or (2) examining the impact of hazards education efforts on awareness and knowledge. As to the first question, the picture painted has been rather bleak (see Covello, 1983; Drabek, 1986; Foster, 1980; Turner et al., 1986). The second question has produced a growing literature with mixed findings. Some of this research has shown little effectiveness (Haas and Trainer, 1974; Roder, 1961; Sorensen, 1983), while other research suggests that disaster education efforts are successful in enhancing prevention and mitigation activities of families (Laska, 1986), and in increasing awareness and preparedness of individuals and families (Faupel, Kelley and Petee, 1992; McKay, 1984; Perry and Greene, 1982; Regulska, 1982; Ruch and Christensen, 1980; Waterstone, 1978).

Given that hazards education seems to be effective, at least under certain circumstances, and given that such education is relatively inexpensive (compared to other mitigation and preparedness measures), we begin with the premise that it is advantageous for local governments to sponsor hazards education programs in their local communities. There is, however, virtually no documentation of what communities across the United States are doing in the way of hazards education. Moreover, we are not aware of *any* research which attempts to explain local governmental efforts at hazards education in the first place.

THEORETICAL APPROACH

This research is part of a broader study examining the impact of the exchange of information and resources between emergency management and city planning agencies on three outcome measures–mitigation, recovery planning, and hazards education. We theorize that the level of hazards education activities should be greater in cities where planning and emergency management agencies are working closely together through the exchange of ideas, resources and expertise. In other contexts, the outcome of such exchange includes changes in perceived legitimacy and status, power, market or supply stability, and other interdependencies among organizations and between them and their environments (Aldrich, 1979). Most studies of inter-organizational coordination in disaster have focused on what factors cause such coordination to occur in the first place. By contrast, virtually no research has been conducted on how new interdependencies of exchange may result in greater effectiveness in program performance. Drabek (1987, p. 169) does address this issue. Referring to the effectiveness of emergency management, he writes that the "singular axiom for emergency management professionals" is the "formation and maintenance" of interagency structures.

Drabek's work, however, focuses only on the coordination role of the emergency management agency itself. We suggest that Drabek's principle can be more broadly applied to the inter-agency relationship between emergency management and city planning. Planning departments are a significant source of poorly tapped local resources to support hazards management generally in at least two ways. First, a close examination of the various activities and functions of a comprehensive hazards management program reveals that local planning offices have a lead role in long term mitigation policies and activities (including zoning authority for environmentally sensitive areas), and it is increasingly clear that these agencies will also have a lead role in long-term recovery processes. Second, planning agencies have routine expertise in areas that could be of great assistance to emergency program managers. For example, planners can provide technical assistance and data for emergency management information systems, such as GIS databases. Planners compile and work with information vital to any city's hazard vulnerability analysis.

Moreover, and specifically relevant to this study, planning departments have much expertise in public involvement and outreach activities. Traditionally, hazards education is a function that is carried out by emergency management agencies. Because of the coordinating role that emergency management agencies play in hazards preparedness and response, it is logical that hazards education is a function carried out by emergency management. Yet, it has been demonstrated that emergency management agencies often lack the resources, training and institutionalized avenues for carrying out hazards education effectively (Labadie, 1984; Caplow, Bahr and Chadwick, 1984). Planning agencies can be a valuable asset to the hazards education agenda of any community, as they are often already involved in educating certain sectors of the public about a variety of issues. Planning works with local builders and business people, for example, regarding zoning and codes issues. Moreover, planning agencies often have institutionalized mechanisms for reaching various audiences through advisory committees, neighborhood development programs, etc. For these reasons, we hypothesize that hazards education activities will be greater in communities with higher levels of interaction between emergency management and planning agencies.

While our study focuses on exchange activities with planning agencies specifically, the more general issue of inter-agency exchange, including exchange with social service agencies, is also at issue. Like planning agencies, social service agencies work with populations which are not as accessible to emergency management agencies. It can also be expected at least, that social service agencies have special skills, such as bilingual versatility, among their personnel to be able to more effectively communicate hazards information to non-English speaking populations. Hence, the benefits associated with exchange with planning offices can also be derived from meaningful exchange with other agencies. With regard to hazards education specifically, the benefit of exchange relationships with social service agencies is especially relevant.

RESEARCH METHODOLOGY

The Sample

The population of cities from which we sampled is comprised of 375 cities surveyed in an earlier national study (Kartez and Lindell, 1987).[1] Survey questionnaires were sent to emergency managers and city planners in all 375 cities. Only the responses from emergency managers are utilized here, as city planners were not surveyed extensively on hazards education. Response rates were exceptionally good, at just under 88 percent, rendering a final sample of 328 cities.

A wide population range is represented in the sample. The smallest community, Barrow, Alaska, reported a population of 2,207 in 1980; no other community in the sample was less than 17,000. Approximately 15 percent of the cities reported populations of less than 25,000. Cities with populations of between 25,000 and 50,000 were the most highly represented, comprising approximately 45 percent of the sample. Another 26 percent are cities between 50,000 and 100,000, and the remaining 19 percent are cities of more than 100,000. The largest city in our sample is Dallas, Texas, with a 1980 population of just over 904,000. Regionally, Western states are most highly represented in our sample, comprising 36 percent of the sample; California alone comprises 21 percent of the sample. Midwestern and Southern states both comprise approximately 29 percent of the cities responding, and Northeastern states comprise only about 6 percent.

Data Collection

Emergency managers were questioned on a variety of hazards-related issues. The variables used for this particular study and their operationalization are discussed below. In addition to the survey, case studies are currently being conducted in several communities which were carefully selected because of the high level of exchange between planning agencies and emergency managers, and for the high levels of mitigation, recovery planning and/or public hazards education activities indicated on the survey responses. As of this time, field visits have been completed in four communities: Bellevue, Washington, Redmond, Washington, Rialto, California and San Bernadino, California. These data are currently being analyzed, and offer some additional insight into the survey responses.

DEPENDENT VARIABLES

Emergency managers were asked to provide information on two aspects of hazards education: (1) to describe how frequently they engaged in any of eight specific hazards educational activities;[2] and (2) those who indicated that they conducted hazards education workshops periodically were further asked to indicate the audiences they reached in these workshops.[3]

The first two dependent variables consist of indices constructed from the eight hazards education variables listed in Note 2. Individual items comprising the indices were Likert scales ranging from 1 (never engage in the activity) to 5 (engage in activity on a monthly basis). Orthomax factoring techniques were employed in order to examine relationships among these variables (Kim and Mueller, 1978a).[4] This procedure yielded two factors which were used as the basis for the construction of our indices. All variables included loaded on the factors with weights ranging from .47 to .74, well above minimal levels suggested (Kim and Mueller, 1978b). Scores on the individual items were multiplied by their factor loadings and then summated to form the indices. The first index, ORALWRIT, is made up of the five variables which simply involve producing written materials or making oral presentations (items 1, 3, 4, 5 and 6 on Note 2; X = 8.78, range = 3.31 to 16.56, sd = 3.11; α = .862). These are comparatively "routine" educational activities for emergency managers. The second index, WORKSHOP, is comprised of more involved and interactive educational activities (items 7 and 8 on Note 2; X = 5.29, range = 1.44 to 7.21, sd = 1.68; α = .681).

These are activities which are not as routinized for most emergency managers. The dependent variable for the third regression, AUDIENCE, is simply a summated index of the number of types of audiences reached by the workshops of those emergency managers who reported conducting workshops as among their educational activities (see Note 3; X = 2.93, range = 0 to 8, sd = 2.50; α = .815).

Independent Variables

A total of seven independent, or predictor, variables are included in this analysis. The variable of theoretical interest in this study (see the theoretical discussion above) is the frequency of interaction between emergency managers and city planners (FREQINT). Emergency managers were asked to indicate how frequently they interacted with representatives from the City Planning Office. Responses were Likert-scaled ranging from (1)–"once a year or less" to (5)–"more than once a week" (X = 4.03; sd = 1.06; Sk = 1.18).

In addition to the level of interaction between emergency management and city planners, we examined the impact of other variables on levels of educational activity. *Disaster experience*, in particular, has been linked to greater disaster preparedness in the sociological literature on the topic (see Drabek, 1986 for a summary of this literature; also Anderson, 1965; Perry and Hirose, 1991; Perry and Lindell, 1990; Mileti et al., 1990; Mulilis and Duval, 1991). We asked emergency managers whether they had experienced a presidentially declared disaster over the past five years. If so, a community was considered to have disaster experience (DISEXP). Those with experience were coded a "1" and those reporting no presidentially declared disasters in their community during the last five years were coded a "0."

In addition to prior disaster experience, *perceived risk* has perhaps been most consistently linked with the adoption of individual and household preparedness and protective actions (Lindell and Barnes, 1986; Sorensen and Mileti, 1987; Mileti et al., 1990). Risk refers to the likelihood that a disaster event will occur sometime in the future. It is reasonable to hypothesize that emergency managers–professionals in their fields–will also be moved to action when they perceive that their communities are subject to hazards risks.

Emergency managers were presented with a list of 11 different types of natural and technological hazards which may or may not pose a risk for their communities. For each of these risks, respondents were asked to indicate whether, for their communities, these potential risks represented: (1) insignificant or no damage potential; (2) minor losses periodically; or (3) substantial risk of catastrophic loss. Responses indicating a *substantial risk* were coded a "1" and no or only minor risks were coded a "0." The scores for all of these variables were then summated (with potential scores ranging from 0 to 11) so as to form an indicator of the *breadth* of risks (HAZRISK) perceived by emergency managers (X = 3.14; sd = 2.03; Sk = 0.39; α = .762).

Other variables were also included in the regressions because of their potential impact on hazards education activities of emergency managers. First, we included a variable measuring the *changing levels of organizational capacity* (with regard to budgets and personnel resources) of emergency management offices to perform all of the various tasks assigned to them (CAPACITY). This is a *relative* variable, ranging from "0" indicating that organizational capacity is decreasing over the past five years, "1" indicating that capacity has not changed, and "2" indicating an increase in organizational capacity (X = 0.86; sd = 0.84; Sk = 0.27). We hypothesized that emergency management offices which had experienced an *increase* in organizational capacity were much more likely to be engaging in hazards education activities than organizations which remained at level or decreasing capacities.

We also hypothesized that emergency management offices with ambitious agendas generally will be much more likely to be involved in hazards education. Managers that merely see their responsibility to coordinate preparedness and response activities are not as likely to be as involved in widespread educational activities as those managers which define their role in a more comprehensive fashion. We asked emergency managers how often they engaged in each of eight planning and preparedness activities.[5] Each of these items was Likert-coded such that a "1" indicated that this activity was conducted less frequently than once every two years, and a "5" indicated that the activity was conducted more frequently than 2-3 times per year. Again, orthomax factoring techniques were employed in order to examine relationships among these variables. This procedure yielded two factors which were used as the basis for the construction of indices. All variables that were included loaded on the factors with weights ranging from .54 to .81. Scores on the individual items were multiplied by their factor loadings and then summated to form the indices. The first index, PREPEXCH, is made up of the four variables which indicate some level of exchange with other agencies. After multiplying responses by their factor loadings, possible scores on this index ranged from 0 to 13.19 (X = 8.28, sd = 2.52, Sk = −.33; α = .648). The second index, PREPSOLO, is comprised of the remaining three preparedness activities which are not inter-agency in nature. Possible scores for this scale ranged from 0 to 11.55 (X = 5.10, sd = 1.71, Sk = .22; α = .722).

Finally, we hypothesized that the population of a community will be directly related to hazards education activities. There are at least two reasons for expecting population to be related to hazards education activities. First, we would expect that larger communities will have larger and more specialized emergency management offices, thereby increasing the likelihood that someone will be specifically assigned the task of education. Both Bellevue, Washington and San Bernadino, California, for example, have full-time hazards education specialists who are housed in the emergency management office. San Bernadino is a relatively large city, with a 1992 population of more than 175,000. Bellevue is somewhat smaller with a 1992 population of 88,580. Cities of much smaller size could not fund such a specialized position. A second reason that we expect population size to be related to hazards education activity is simply that larger cities are more likely to pose a greater *demand* from various sectors of the community for hazards education.

The Regressions

A total of three regressions were performed, examining the impact of the predictor variables on ORALWRIT, WORKSHOP, and AUDIENCE, respectively (Tables 1, 2, and 3). Correlations of all the variables used in the regressions revealed that the highest correlation between the independent variables is .451 (between PREPEXCH and PREPSOLO), indicating a lack of multi-colinearity among the variables.[6]

TABLE 1. Factors Affecting the Frequency of Oral and Written Hazards Education Activities Conducted by Emergency Managers (Reported by Emergency Managers)

Variable	Unstandardized Coefficient (b)	Standardized Coefficient (β)	Standard Error (SE)
FREQINT	.235	.083	.169
DISEXP	.490	.078	.377
HAZRISK	.131	.086	.092
CAPACITY	.179	.048	.220
PREPEXCH	.445[a]	.364	.083
PREPSOLO	.225	.122	.119
POP80	.000	.046	.000

Adjusted $R^2 = .251$ $F = 11.789$[a]
[a]$p < .001$
[b]$p < .01$
[c]$p < .05$

TABLE 2. Factors Affecting the Frequency of Hazards Education Workshops Conducted by Emergency Managers (Reported by Emergency Managers)

Variable	Unstandardized Coefficient (b)	Standardized Coefficient (β)	Standard Error (SE)
FREQINT	.204[c]	.112	.115
DISEXP	.276	.068	.257
HAZRISK	.185[b]	.186	.063
CAPACITY	.145	.060	.150
PREPEXCH	.169[b]	.214	.056
PREPSOLO	.134	.113	.081
POP80	.000	.019	.000

Adjusted $R^2 = .171$ $F = 7.638$[a]
[a]$p < .001$
[b]$p < .01$
[c]$p < .05$

Table 1 examines the impact of our predictor variables on the level of oral and written hazards education activities by emergency managers while controlling for all other variables. Overall, the model accounts for more than 25 percent of the variance; however,

TABLE 3. Factors Affecting the Breadth of Hazards Education Audiences by Emergency Managers (Reported by Emergency Managers)

Variable	Unstandardized Coefficient (b)	Standardized Coefficient (β)	Standard Error (SE)
FREQINT	.351[c]	.156	.137
DISEXP	.311	.062	.306
HAZRISK	.199[b]	.163	.075
CAPACITY	.237	.080	.179
PREPEXCH	.290[a]	.298	.067
PREPSOLO	.117	.080	.097
POP80	.000	−.019	.000

Adjusted $R^2 = .223$ $F = 10.283$[a]
[a]$p < .001$
[b]$p < .01$
[c]$p < .05$

the only single predictor that significantly affects the level of oral and written educational activities is PREPEXCH, which is the frequency of inter-agency preparedness activities by emergency managers.

These results are not that surprising since *most* emergency managers are involved in oral and written hazards education activities. Oral and written forms of hazards education, such as publishing brochures and speaking to schools and community groups, is routine for most emergency managers. Hence, interaction with city planning offices does not particularly enhance this type of hazards education activity, which is already going on anyway. The only variable that *does* significantly affect oral and written hazards education is the frequency of inter-agency preparedness activities that emergency managers engage in (see Note 5). We suspect that this relationship may be spurious. That is, there is probably nothing inherent to these inter-agency preparedness activities that promotes greater levels of hazards education, but rather, emergency management organizations which go to the effort of being inter-departmentally involved are probably also organizations which will take more seriously their role as hazards educators. These inter-agency activities represent a substantially greater commitment to the emergency preparedness process than preparedness activities which are not inter-agency in scope (PREPSOLO), and which are much more routine in nature.

Unlike producing written and oral materials, conducting interactive workshops requires an extensive amount of planning and investment of comparably greater investments of time and resources. Table 2 reveals that while our predictor variables, collectively, account for less of the variation in workshop activity (about 17%), three of the variables in the model are significant.

The frequency of interaction with city planners *is* a significant predictor of hazards education workshops, as is the frequency of inter-agency preparedness activities. In addition, the number of perceived hazards risks is a significant predictor of workshop activity. The latter finding is interesting because hazards workshops allow for a much more thorough treatment of multiple hazards issues. They are typically interactive in nature, thereby providing a forum for presentation of complex and multi-faceted information that is required for a broad range of hazards risks.

The number of *hazards audiences* refers to the breadth of exposure that emergency managers attempt in their workshop activities, regardless of the frequency with which they engage in these activities. Overall, the model accounts for just over 22% of the variance.

As with the hazards education activities, the level of inter-agency preparedness activity is significantly and directly related to breadth of hazards audiences targeted for educational workshops. Similarly, interaction with city planners increases the breadth of audiences targeted. These relationships suggest that inter-agency activity, and particularly exchange activities with city planning, may alert emergency management organizations to or provide them much better access to a broader constituency for hazards education activities, a constituency not normally part of their routine interactive network (e.g., builders and contractors or possibly even business owners). In addition, both perceived hazards risks and recent disaster experience are related to the number of types of hazards audiences targeted. Again, it appears that these experiences and perceptions underscore the importance of a broadly knowledgeable population. One of our respondents in Bellevue captured an orientation that seems to be operative among those for whom the possibility of hazardous events is salient: "If you can't get the community prepared for itself, it will increase the overwhelming demand for resources."

IMPLICATIONS

The findings presented here suggest, first, that emergency managers are conscientiously involved in what might be called "traditional" hazards educational activities (see Note 2). A strong majority of the emergency managers in our sample were involved in traditional forms of information distribution such as producing and distributing brochures, seeking media coverage of hazards issues, speaking to community groups and schools, etc. Even more encouraging, nearly three-fourths (72%) indicated that they engaged in at least four (4) of these activities on a regular basis. More extensive educational activities requiring greater commitment of time and resources, such as workshops and special hazards events in the community, are less frequently engaged in, however. Prior research (Faupel, Kelley and Petee, 1992) suggests that such educational efforts do pay off by way of increased individual and household preparedness for disaster events. Our data thus suggest that emergency managers need to focus more effort on interactive-style educational programs in the future.

Frequency of interaction with planning departments significantly (though modestly) predicts both the likelihood of promoting hazards education workshops and the number of audiences reached, when controlling for other variables. Interaction with planning does *not* impact on the likelihood of the more traditional oral and written hazards education activities. Nevertheless, these data suggest to us that, indeed, hazards education benefits from the interface between emergency management and city planning departments. Emergency management organizations which are interacting on a regular basis with planning departments are clearly more committed to creative and resource-intensive workshop-type activities; and more committed to reaching a broader variety of audiences for their educational activities. It is also worthwhile pointing out again that communities which are confronted with numerous hazards risks tend to be more likely to engage in workshop activities, and to reach a wider audience than those communities with fewer risks; and that communities with recent disaster experience also reach a wider audience. It would appear, therefore, that exposure to natural and technological hazards, combined with interaction with city planning, promotes a stronger commitment to hazards education beyond routine, traditional activities.

These findings suggest that systematic, structured interaction between planning, emergency management, and other hazards-relevant departments of city and county government, including social service and relief agencies, should contribute substantially to effective hazards education in local communities. Bellevue, Washington has established such a structure, called the "Emergency Operations Board" consisting of the Deputy City Manager, the city attorney, the fire and police chiefs, and heads of Community Development, Finance, Human Resources, Parks, Planning, Transportation and Utilities departments. This board deliberates policy recommendations made by a lower-level "Emergency Management Committee" consisting of representatives of all of the hazards-relevant departments of city government. After deliberation, the Emergency Operations Board then makes policy recommendations to City Council. This procedure has the dual advantage of involving all department directors in hazards policy, thereby encouraging more inter-departmental involvement; and of hazards policy recommendations having a high level, and consensus endorsement, before going before city council. Hazards issues generally, including hazards education, have high visibility in the city of Bellevue.

Exposure to hazards risks clearly contributes to greater efforts at hazards education. Some communities, however, are not waiting for disaster to strike. These communities are using the experiences of other communities in disasters as lessons in how they can better prepare and respond. Bellevue, Washington routinely sends employees in various departments of city government to disaster sites all around the country to learn what problems their counterparts in these cities faced in a disaster situation. It is the goal of Bellevue officials to send representatives from every relevant department of city government to a community victimized by disaster to learn from the experiences of counterpart agencies in these communities. San Bernadino and Rialto, California also visit disaster sites, though on a less systematic basis. The result of this commitment on the part of these city governments is not only a better informed staff, but over time, these cities are raising their awareness of the threat of disaster and what they need to be doing to prepare for hazards in their communities. Communities can benefit from the disaster experience of other communities in this way.

Moreover, because effective, workshop-type hazards education is so labor intensive, there are real constraints on how much an emergency management department can do working on its own. The City of San Bernadino has recognized the value of working jointly with other organizations and groups by establishing a "target population" approach to hazards education in an effort to respond to educational needs as efficiently as possible. The Emergency Manager's office identifies one or more population sectors to target for a given year. One year it was the business community; another year it was residents living in trailer parks; another year it was the disabled. Once identified, the participation of leaders within these target populations is solicited to develop and carry out an educational agenda. Hence, rather than carrying the entire burden for hazards education, the office of the emergency manager was equipping others to carry out the educational process. While, to our knowledge, social service agencies were not directly involved in this process, their potential value in identifying target populations and in assisting in communicating this information to certain populations is obvious. This program has met with mixed success in San Bernadino, but is suggestive of an approach to hazards education that can reach more people in a substantial manner, beyond the traditional one-time dissemination of brochures and other written and oral information.

Finally, and especially relevant to many readers, close working relationships with other agencies, particularly social service agencies, can facilitate this process considerably. Such relationships benefit both emergency management and social service delivery agencies. Emergency management benefits because Departments of Human Resources and similar agencies have daily contact with a sector of the population which is typically difficult to reach through traditional hazards education approaches (e.g., see Faupel, Kelley and Petee, 1992). With effective working relationships with emergency managers, these departments can be a valuable ally in dissemination of hazards information to some of the more marginal, but most vulnerable, segments of a community's population. Social service agencies benefit in this exchange because while these organizations have mandates to respond to human suffering and provide aid and relief to (typically) marginal populations, they are organized to deliver these services under normal, non-disaster conditions. In many communities, these agencies are severely limited in their ability to reach these residents. Effective working relationships with emergency management provides valuable knowledge and understanding of the obstacles *and* opportunities for service delivery in a greatly altered community structure which comprises a new and, for some, uncharted environment in which they must work. More important, such working relationships plug social service delivery agencies into the emergency preparedness and response network. Hence, these agencies can more effectively be educating, equipping, and preparing their clients for potential disaster through the access that they have to the resources of the emergency preparedness and response system.

NOTES

1. This population of cities was used so as to allow for longitudinal analysis. The present study does not make use of the longitudinal data.

2. The eight educational activities were:

   *1. Distribute hazard education or preparedness brochures to the public. (81.5%)**

   2. Conduct community special events such as emergency preparedness day. (53.6%)

   3. Seek local news media coverage of hazards management topics. (70.4%)

   4. Publish information for citizens on emergency preparedness or home mitigation in local phone directory or newspaper. (66.6%)

   5. Speak about hazards management to community groups. (79.6%)

   6. Speak about hazards management in local schools. (67.9%)

   7. Conduct how-to workshops for small businesses on recovery or mitigation. (27.7%)

   8. Conduct other workshops on preparedness, mitigation or recovery. (47.7%)

   ****Percentage of respondents who indicated this activity on at least an annual basis.***

3. Audiences identified were: *general public (58.3%), senior citizens (42.3%), school teachers (40.7%), health care professionals (40.7%), business owners (38.6%), news media professionals (24.7%), handicapped or other special populations (22.8%), contractors/builders (8.3%), and "other" (16.7%).*

4. Orthomax factoring procedures are ordinarily used for interval level data with a normal distribution. There is a precedent, however, in using these procedures for ordinal level data when the ordinal categories are approximately equal and when there is a normal distribution across the categories. The variables comprising these factors consist of approximately equal categories ("Never," "Less than Annually," "Annually," "A Few Times a Year" and "Monthly"). Moreover, the distribution across these categories is normal (Sk < 1.00 for all variables).

5. Preparedness activities involving some level of exchange with other agencies (PREPEXCH) included: *multi-department emergency exercises, interdepartmental emergency management committee meetings, meetings with a Title-III LEPC, and coordination meetings with the county emergency manager.* Preparedness activities *not* involving exchange with other agencies (PREPSOLO) included: *update of the basic disaster plan, updates of each department's SOP or annexes, and review of emergency roles and procedures with city council.* Two items on these scales merit some brief discussion. First, "LEPC" refers to the Local Emergency Planning Committee, a multi-agency, multi-interest emergency planning body for local government which is required by the Emergency Planning and Community Right-to-Know Act of 1986, and jointly administered by the Federal Emergency Management Agency and the Environmental Protection Agency. The committees are mandated to include local public agencies, industrial facility personnel and community groups in planning for toxic chemical disasters. In some communities, the LEPC mandate represents a major broadening of the emergency management audience while in others it may be dominated by fire department personnel and industrial facility employees. Second, it might be noted that updating each department's SOP is, in fact, interagency in nature. However, it loaded strongly on the PREPSOLO factor (.78). This is understandable, since these departmental updates are a routine part of the emergency planning process in many if not most cities.

6. The complete correlation matrix is available from the lead author on request. PREPEXCH and PREPSOLO also had the highest variance inflation factors of 1.38 and 1.28 respectively, again indicating that multi-colinearity is not a factor in these models.

REFERENCES

Aldrich, H. 1979. *Organizations and Environment.* Englewood Cliffs, NJ: Prentice-Hall.

Anderson, W. 1965. *Some Observations on a Disaster Subculture: The Organizational Response of Cincinnati, Ohio to the 1964 Flood.* Disaster Research Center Report #6. Columbus, OH: The Ohio State University.

Caplow, T., H. Bahr, and B. Chadwick. 1984. *Analysis of the Readiness of Local Communities for Integrated Emergency Management Planning*. Final Report to the Federal Emergency Management Agency. Washington, D.C.: U.S. Government Printing Office.

Covello, V. 1983. "The perception of technological risks: a literature review." *Technological Forecasting and Social Change* 23: 285-297.

Drabek, Thomas. 1986. *Human System Responses to Disaster: An Inventory of Sociological Findings*. New York: Springer-Verlag.

______. 1987. *The Professional Emergency Manager*. Boulder, CO: Institute of Behavioral Science, University of Colorado.

Faupel, Charles E., Susan P. Kelley and Thomas Petee. 1992. "The impact of disaster education on household preparedness for Hurricane Hugo." *International Journal of Mass Emergencies and Disasters*. 10,1:5-24.

Foster, H. 1980. *Disaster Planning*. New York: Springer-Verlag.

Haas, J. and P. Trainer. 1974. "Effectiveness of tsunami warning systems in selected coastal towns in Alaska." Rome: Proceedings of the Fifth World Conference on Earthquake Engineering.

Kartez, Jack and Michael Lindell. 1987. "Planning for uncertainty: the case of local disaster planning." *Journal of the American Planning Association* 53,4:487-498.

Kim, Jae-On and Charles W. Mueller. 1978a. *Introduction to Factor Analysis: What it is and How to do it*. Beverly Hills, CA: Sage Publications.

_____ 1978b. *Factor Analysis: Statistical Methods and Practical Issues*. Beverly Hills, CA: Sage Publications.

Labadie, J. 1984. "Problems in local emergency management." *Environmental Management* 8:489-494.

Laska, Shirley. 1986. "Involving homeowners in flood mitigation." *Journal of the American Planning Association*. 52:452-466.

Lindell, M. and V. Barnes. 1986. "Protective response to technological emergency: risk perception and behavioral intention." *Nuclear Safety* 27:457-467.

McKay, J. 1984. "Community response to hazard information." *Disasters* 8,2:118-123.

Mileti, D.S., C. Fitzpatrick, and B.C. Farhar. 1990. *Risk Communication and Public Response to the Parkfield Earthquake Prediction Experiment*. Final Report to the National Science Foundation. Fort Collins: Hazards Assessment Laboratory and Department of Sociology, Colorado State University.

Mulilis, J.-P. and T.S. Duval. 1991. "The impact of nearby earthquakes on individual earthquake preparedness." Paper presented at the UCLA International Conference on the Impact of Natural Disasters, Los Angeles, July 9-12.

Perry, R. and H. Hirose. 1991. *Volcano Management in the United States and Japan*. Greenwich, CT: JAI Press.

Perry R. and M. Lindell. 1990. "Predicting long term adjustment to volcano hazard." *International Journal of Mass Emergencies and Disasters*. 8:117-136.

Perry, Ronald W. and Marjorie Greene. 1982. "The role of ethnicity in the emergency decision-making process." *Sociological Inquiry* 52,4:306-334.

Regulska, Joanna. 1982. "Public awareness programs for natural hazards." Pp. 36-70 in Thomas F. Saarinen (ed.), *Perspectives on Increasing Hazard Awareness*. Boulder, CO: Institute for Behavioral Science, University of Colorado.

Roder, W. 1961. "Attitude and knowledge on the Topeka flood plain." Pp. 62-92 in Gilbert F. White (ed.), *Papers on Flood Problems*. Chicago: Department of Geography, University of Chicago.

Ruch, Carlton E. and L. Christensen. 1980. "Hurricane message enhancement." College Station, TX: Sea Grant College Program, Texas A&M University.

Sorensen, John H. 1983. "Knowing how to behave under the threat of disaster: can it be explained?" *Environment and Behavior* 15,4:438-457.

Sorensen, J. and D. Mileti. 1987. "Programs that encourage the adoption of precautions against natural hazards." In N. Weinstein (ed.), *Taking Care*. Cambridge: Cambridge University Press.

Turner, Ralph H., Joanne M. Nigg and Denise H. Paz. *Waiting for Disaster: Earthquake Watch in California*. Berkeley, CA: University of California Press.

Waterstone, Marvin. 1978. "Hazard mitigation behavior of urban flood plain residents." Natural Hazards Research Working Paper #35. Boulder, CO: Institute of Behavioral Science, University of Colorado.

Index

Page numbers in italics indicate figures; page numbers followed by t indicate tables.